GET A WHIFF OF THIS

Perfumes (fragrances) - the Invisible Chemical Poisons

By

Connie Pitts

Edited By

Stephanee Killen

© 2003 by Connie Pitts. All rights reserved.

No part of this book may be reproduced, stored in a retrieval system, or transmitted by any means, electronic, mechanical, photocopying, recording, or otherwise, without written permission from the author.

ISBN: 1-4140-0844-9 (e-book)
ISBN: 1-4140-0845-7 (Paperback)
ISBN: 1-4140-0846-5 (Dust Jacket)

Library of Congress Control Number: 2003096854

This book is printed on acid free paper.

Printed in the United States of America
Bloomington, IN

1stBooks – rev. 10/01/03

I dedicate this book to the millions of people who suffer from chemically induced illnesses and to the countless people who have worked diligently towards change.

To my family.

TABLE OF CONTENTS

FOREWORD vii
PREFACE xiii
ACKNOWLEDGMENTS xv
INTRODUCTION xvii
AN OVERALL UNVEILING OF FRAGRANCE FACTS xix
HOW PERFUMES HAVE AFFECTED MY LIFE (My Story)
.... xxiii
CHAPTER 1 PERFUMES AND THE CANCER CONNECTION
.... 1

   Cosmetics Linked to the Causes of Breast Cancer and Fatal Breast Cancer... 3

   Cancer Prevention Coalition and Environmental Health Network . 9

CHAPTER 2 THE PETITION FILED AGAINST THE U.S. FDA
.... 13

   The Environmental Health Network (EHN) 15

   Review the Chemical Analysis of Calvin Klein's Eternity Eau De Parfum 20

   Responses to the Petition 24

   Responding to the Petition 41

CHAPTER 3 PERFUMES POSE SERIOUS HEALTH RISKS 43

   Health Risks from Perfumes: 46

   Making Sense of Scents 52

   Fragrance Chemicals as Toxic Substances.............................. 55

   Synthetic Musk Linked to Environmental Risks..................... 58

CHAPTER 4 ANDERSON LABORATORIES 63

   Acute Toxic Effects of Fragrance Products 65

   Toxic Effects of Air Freshener Emissions 67

CHAPTER 5 ABSTRACT **69**
  Abstract of Article on Dana Perfume Co. 71
CHAPTER 6 HALIFAX, NOVA SCOTIA OUTLAWS PERFUMES THE REAL FACTS **73**
  Note from Nova Scotia: Perfume Stinks 75
  The "REAL" Facts the Fragrance Industry Doesn't Want You to Know 76
CHAPTER 7 SCENTED CANDLES – THE REAL DIRT **83**
  Dangers of Fragranced Candles 85
  Candles, Toxic Emissions, and Property Damage 88
CHAPTER 8 THE EFFECTS OF CHEMICALS ON WOMEN AND CHILDREN MONEY RULES **91**
  Chemicals Pose a Higher Risk for Females 93
  Environmental Research Foundation MONEY RULES 95
CHAPTER 9 C.T.F.A. **97**
  Cosmetic, Toiletry, and Fragrance Association 99
CHAPTER 10 GOVERNMENT KNOWLEDGE **101**
  Safe Notification Information for Fragrances [SNIFF] 103
  Federal Aviation Administration (FAA) 105
  Governor Bush's Proclamation 107
  To Report Adverse Health Effects of Fragrances 109
  What the U.S. Government [FDA] Is Doing About It 111
CHAPTER 11 WEBSITES SAFER PRODUCTS **115**
  Informative Websites: 117
  Safer Products 118
CONCLUSION **122**
ADDITIONAL BOOKS OF INTEREST **125**
APPENDIX **127**
RESOURCES **130**

FOREWORD

Brother, here we go again . . .

This is actually the refrain from an old song, which became a slogan in my family when challenging times came back in a sort of re-circulating pattern. Not much more than a memory fragment, but it is sufficient. It could be the subtitle for this book, *GET A WHIFF OF THIS*. Connie Pitts is giving us the story of perfume—or more comprehensively, of fragrance. She provides the human poisoning story and the backup data, which gives credibility to an unlikely tale (unless you have been there, along with a growing number of Americans). This data shows us just how much is already known on the subject of poisons in fragrances. The surprise is that with so much already in the public arena, the possibility of perfume poisoning is completely unknown to so many.

Although fragrances are the center of this contentious issue, we have heard the story hundreds of times on our phone about many different products. It could be the story of carpets, air fresheners, fabric softeners, pesticides, felt tip markers, or formaldehyde. Asbestos, lead, tobacco, mercury and PCB, and dioxin and hormone disruptors belong in the same category. The list is as long as you want to make it. Love Canal is not a proud memory. As a society, we have been through this fight over and over and when we read a book such as *GET A WHIFF OF THIS,* we learn, to our sorrow, how heavily the mechanisms for change are stacked against the small guy.

Scores of individuals have failed to win when the issue was asbestos exposure or lead poisoning, each of which is now considered a no-brainer. There was enough information in the 1930s to indicate the future of lead in gasoline. After untold damage, steps were taken to get it out. We knew sufficient information when I was in school to institute precautionary steps concerning the mass production of asbestos-containing products and the same is true of tobacco. Not until late in the century were these issues prominent enough to cause formal action. Most of the other chemical issues have yet to be seriously examined and resolved. Until the situation is in our neighborhood, we tend to expect that a government safety net combined with human decency are enough to protect us. Let us look.

Friends, Family, and Others
Brother, here we go again. The story is always the same. An individual suffers from health problems following exposure to some product or chemical, which as consumers we assume is suitable for human use. The health complaints seem to be unusual, or even bizarre, and are therefore suspect in the eyes of friends, relations, and coworkers. Often, the same message from a third party "expert" is needed to make the obvious real to the closest associates.

The symptoms are denied by the employer (if job related). We have heard of some noteworthy exceptions, but the impulse to hide from a potentially costly challenge is strong. Workers compensation is expensive.

Industry
Here we go again. About industry, we have sometimes heard that the manufacturer responded that this was the very first and only complaint ever received. Being in the middle of the battle at the time, we knew that was not the case. Manufacturers are often very hard to contact. The phone number on the box is not always in service. The address may be incorrect. The help line and the hold line are sometimes interchangeable.

The manufacturer of most products is at liberty to share information concerning a product or not. A material safety data sheet (MSDS) may be available or not. The desired information may be on the MSDS or not. The health test data may exist or not.

Manufacturers of many consumer items are in a strange position. If they test a product for possible health effects and find some bad news, it is reportable. If they fail to test the product, there is nothing to report, and that is just fine with the regulatory agencies. Self-regulation under these circumstances is a non-starter. Needless to say, careful testing is unusual. The positive step would be to put the burden of proof on industry with reports to a non-government watchdog pack.

Medicine
The reports of a new syndrome are frequently rejected by the medical profession. The physicians of this country have very good memories,

but our experience is that they are unwilling to consider ideas, which did not originate in their school days. They are almost universally ignorant concerning poisoning by chemicals and chemical mixtures. A positive step would be to add environmental toxic exposures to the curriculum.

Local Health Department
Somehow, in this abstract scenario, the exposure remains outside the jurisdiction of the local health department. Often, this is because there are no established limits for acceptable air contamination. Or else, as in the case of fragrances, the levels are established for single chemical exposure and do not apply to the multi-chemical mix of real life. The budget is always limited, and we have a tendency to shoot the messenger. This does not make for good communication.

There are also informal agency barriers in the form of tradition and attitude, which prevent general recognition of the validity of these unwelcome (sometimes budget busting) complaints.

This attitude barrier was mind blowing when Anderson Laboratories conducted an indoor air health study of a school building. We toured the school looking at the details of how it was built, cleaned, maintained, and furnished. We interviewed faculty and staff members and heard multiple reports about health problems associated with their hours working in the building. We made the usual measurements, and as a final precaution to test our impression that the building was indeed very sick, we took several large air samples back to our laboratory. Using a standardized test method, we found that the animals breathing air collected outside the building showed no change in their excellent health status. The animals breathing air from the kindergarten room were immediately showing signs of toxic chemical exposure, and one animal died within fifteen minutes—a very unusual and severe indication of trouble.

In a follow-up meeting of parents, staff, and students, we explained our findings, followed by a state health officer who agreed that the building needed immediate attention. After the meeting, he came up to me and said, "I study this school every year. It is a very bad building, but they never do anything." He showed me his stack of reports, each one a copy of the previous year suggesting that some remedial action might be beneficial. Then he added, "But you should never have mentioned that mouse." When asked why, he replied, *"People might get upset."* Indeed, the parents *did* get upset, primarily because the data had been minimized for years by an official who felt that his job was to protect his agency from controversy rather than to protect the youngest children from a preventable toxic exposure. (They also got angry much to the benefit of the school.)

Federal Agencies

Here we go again. When health problems associated with commercial products are presented to federal agencies, they frequently use the excuse that they are unable to find published literature concerning the health effects of the product. They have actually said, "No published data, no problem." Right? The validity of this logic is right up there with tobacco junk science and should never be tolerated.

It is true that for product toxicity issues, scientific data is generally not available. This is to be expected: there is no published research in these areas because there has been no federal money to fund the research—and no requirement for industry to do it either.

We see from the Eternity Petition that even when there is data, and when the petitioners follow the rules to the letter and a thousand people endorse the complaint, the federal agency chooses not to comply with its own procedures. This situation is stupid but real.

Thousands of new chemicals hit the market every year with no safety data. Without data of some valid sort (one million happy users is not valid data), no agency can take action in any direction. The positive step would be to establish a mechanism (and funding), which would allow them to briefly evaluate recurrent health claims with carefully designed survey studies. The *"Yes, but . . ."* is that such work must be performed without an external agenda. Sadly, the "agenda" directs the research and the sponsor by choosing the details of the study.

Using another approach, federal agencies often claim lack of jurisdiction as a reason for being uninvolved. This is often valid; however, when there is a popular cause, we note a proliferation of agencies, which, by creative interpretation of the wording of their charters, find a way to be involved. It must be noted that many government agencies have had the experience of being seen as too forceful with respect to some not so popular issue. The control point, as always, is money. Money comes from congress and what congress delivers congress can also take away. And they do. Industry pressure on congressional funding is said to work well. And if an agency is considered to be naughty, the budget may be cut for more than the "offending project." Talking with government workers teaches us that the punitive budget cut is something that lasts in the memory for a long time. It works well.

What is broke here? Everything. The system is corrupt, and no easy fix will emerge.

Back to Perfume

Brother, here we go again. With all of this in mind, this story of exposure and its consequences is ugly but predictable. The part that cannot be predicted is how soon this issue will blow up.

We already know enough now to take strong steps to limit the mass marketing of dangerous fragrance products. What we know has all been accomplished without the help of health departments, industry, or the federal government. The human experimentation has been completed using millions of individuals without their informed consent. Too bad the data collection by the industry has been ignored. Even so, epidemiology is starting to show up. We know that a very large percentage of the general population reports health effects following fragrance exposure. Some factory workers have filed complaints due to fragrance pollution in the plant. In an inspired move, individuals have petitioned for a warning on the label of a carcinogen-containing perfume. Medicine now acknowledges the links between perfume and human asthma (a fatal disease) in repeated publications. Toxicology studies, which demonstrate irritation, asthma, and neurotoxicity, have been published without challenge. More is on the way. (As I write, in the laboratory, we are studying the neurotoxicity of a cube of solid air freshener, which measures 1/4 inch on a side.) There is no question about the potency of these products.

Chemistry tells us a story of carcinogens, irritants, asthma triggers, and neurotoxins. Books by Connie Pitts and Louise Kosta focus entirely on fragrances, and newspapers are starting to see the story. We have legal precedent of assault by perfumed products and whole communities are agreeing to restrictions concerning fragrances in public places.

We know enough, and it is summarized in *GET A WHIFF OF THIS*. Perhaps it is time to get angry.

Rosalind C. Anderson, Ph.D.

PREFACE

Perfumes were once derived from natural sources, such as wild flowers, plants, and diluted animal secretions. Musk was derived from the gland of the genitalia of the male musk deer. After World War II, synthetic chemicals were discovered, and they were much cheaper and easier to use for creating fragrances. Throughout the last fifty years, much has changed in perfume making, particularly since the 70s and early 1980s. Due to *Trade Secret* laws, most people are not aware of what's really in these products.

The fragrance industry certainly portrays their products as benign, with advertisements publicizing perfumes and other *scented* goods as fresh, clean, alluring, sexy, and pure, often including a bouquet of flowers in the background. The truth is that perfumes contain a large number of harmful substances. Few perfume chemicals are safety tested. Although fragrances fall under the jurisdiction of the FDA, they are not regulated.

This book will supply information you have a right to know. You will finally learn the truth, empowering yourself to utilize wise decisions regarding purchasing personal care products while enhancing your understanding of your health and the health of those around you.

It's unlikely that you will learn what I'm about to share from newspapers or television media due to advertising dollar revenues.

What you are about to learn is not pretty.

I've included my own personal story, which includes additional evidence. I am a *former* user of numerous fragranced products.

ACKNOWLEDGMENTS

I would like to extend special thanks to the following people:

Betty Bridges, RN, head of the Fragranced Products Information Network, for her encouragement, willingness to answer my numerous questions, and for giving me permission to share her work.

Barbara Wilke, President of the Environmental Health Network of California, for her willingness to keep me continually updated with information, for answering many of my questions, and for giving me permission to share her work.

James W. Coleman, Ph.D., President/CEO of the Cancer Research Center of America, Inc., for giving me permission to share his work, guidelines to follow, reviewing my manuscript, teaching me computer savvy, and having confidence in me. I will always be grateful for his countless hours of generous help.

Amy Marsh, former President of the Environmental Health Network, Larkspur, California, for granting me permission to share her letters written to the FDA.

Julius Anderson, M.D., Ph.D., Vice President, Anderson Laboratories, Inc. and Rosalind C. Anderson, Ph.D., Anderson Laboratories, Inc., for their willingness to review my manuscript for accuracy pertaining to their studies and for giving me permission to share their work.

Richard H. Conrad, Ph.D., Biochemist, for his patience when I've called him in the morning hours.

Cathy Flanders, for giving me permission to share her work and for being at the forefront in regards to bringing awareness to the dangers of scented candles.

Maria Pellerano, Associate Director, Environmental Research Foundation, Rachel's Environment & Health News, for giving me permission to use their material.

Sandra L. Moser, Citizens for A Safe Learning Environment, for giving me permission to share her writing.

To everyone who wrote letters to the U.S. FDA in support of the petition to declare Calvin Klein's Eternity eau de parfum misbranded.

I also wish to thank Hollie Hoffman, Janine Ridings, Kathleen Houghton, Linda Conrad, Helle Kongevang, Lynn Lawson, and Terri Lindberg for their unwavering support and friendship.

Thanks to Gregory Squires for designing a striking book cover illustration.

INTRODUCTION

Most people are aware of the toxic effects of tobacco smoke. In recent years, there has also been increased publicity regarding toxic molds and pesticides. Much like pesticides, perfumes contain neurotoxins, which are chemicals that poison the nervous system. But many people are still in the dark when it comes to the serious health risks related to exposures from perfumes, colognes, and other *scented* products, most often referred to as fragrances. Due to an extreme lack of media attention, I felt that a book targeting unsuspecting consumers is long overdue.

Not everyone owns a computer, nor do the vast majority of people go online in order to investigate perfumes. Unfortunately, I am one of many who have done so. When perfumes started making me seriously ill, I wanted to know if it was simply me or if there was something possibly amiss with perfumes. Much of the information was easily obtainable via the Internet. What I learned was quite shocking!

Eventually sickened by my own perfume and second-hand exposures from other people's fragrances, my illness led me to search for answers. My health continued to plummet with each perfume exposure, and I had begun to have reactions to other products containing synthetic fragrances. I conducted a search and joined a Listserv group, the FPIN (Fragranced Products Information Network). Finally, I would see exactly what was in these products that caused millions of people serious illnesses—ranging from life-threatening asthma, chronic migraines and fatigue, to poor concentration, combative behavior, and heart arrhythmias, to name some of the more common symptoms. For the first time, I read about Multiple Chemical Sensitivities (MCS). MCS has become an epidemic in the United States. MCS is defined by many *expert* doctors as when a person suffers serious, adverse health effects to low levels of toxic and hazardous chemicals, although there is not a case definition, due to lack of Congressional support. Many fragrance chemicals can act as sensitizers, causing immune system damage so that you become allergic to the chemical. [13]

I've corresponded with many new friends, including experts in the field of health, pioneer activists, and researchers. I spent two years trying to gain the interest of law firms in hopes of bringing forth much needed public awareness, although my efforts seemed futile.

Fragrance chemicals do not end with a bottle of perfume or cologne. They can be found in common items such as hair care products, hairsprays, deodorants, body lotions, sunscreens, aftershaves, shaving gels, as well as laundry detergents, fabric softeners, dryer sheets, scented plug-ins, scented candles, potpourri, alleged air *fresheners,* most cleaning products, anti-bacterial creams, disinfectants, magazines, and even in trash bags and pesticides—and the list goes on.

The fragrance industry does not have to divulge their product's contents to the FDA due to an old and outdated adage called Trade Secret. Considering the numerous imitation perfumes, Trade Secret seems absurd. Doctors cannot easily obtain information regarding the ingredients in scented products, even if they feel it is causing illness.

I'm sharing my story so that people may understand how synthetic fragrances can affect a person's life, altering their lifestyle in a way that I feel is inhumane, while also affecting family members and friends. Throughout the last few years, I started clipping newspaper articles in reference to perfumes, air fresheners, and colognes. Illnesses from exposures to these products are on the rise. My story includes information regarding Halifax, Nova Scotia where perfumes and other artificially scented products have been outlawed in most public buildings; the efforts of one Congresswoman, Janice Schakowsky, who introduced the SNIFF Bill HR 1947 (Safe Notification Information For Fragrances) to no avail; and a petition filed against the FDA in 1999 to declare a popular perfume misbranded.

I'd like to share some of the information I've presented to lawyers. You may wish to share the evidence with your health care provider or doctor. The ignorance within our health establishment, in this country, is almost inconceivable. If thousands of average people such as myself could obtain scientific and medical journals regarding the health risks of perfumes—information that most mainstream doctors have never seen—then something is wrong with this picture.

We have been duped by an industry that has no regard for human health or our environment and a government that condones it.

AN OVERALL UNVEILING OF FRAGRANCE FACTS

Many chemicals used to make perfumes and other scented products are listed on the Environmental Protection Agency's (EPA) **Hazardous Waste List.** [1]

Approximately 95% of chemicals used in fragrances are synthetic compounds derived from petroleum. They include **benzene** derivatives, **aldehydes,** and many other known toxins and **sensitizers**, which are capable of causing cancer, central nervous system (CNS) disorders, birth defects, and allergic reactions. – Report by the Committee on Science & Technology. "Neurotoxins: At Home and the Workplace." U.S. House of Representatives, Sept. 16, 1986. (Report 99-827)

There are many neurological disorders, including Multiple Sclerosis, Lupus, Alzheimer's, and Parkinson's Disease. Dyslexia is a neurological dysfunction, as well as Sudden Infant Death Syndrome (SIDS). Could neurotoxic chemicals in fragranced detergents, fabric softeners, or dryer sheets be causing the neurological breakdown? [2] Chloroform was found in tests of fabric softeners. (**EPA's** 1991 study.) [3] A room containing an air freshener has high levels of p-dichlorobenzene (a carcinogen) and ethanol. [3]

According to recent information from the National Institute of Health, 26.3 million Americans have been diagnosed with asthma. Those numbers continue to rise at alarmingly high rates. Seventy-two percent of asthmatics report that fragrances trigger their asthma. According to a report by the CDC's National Center for Health Statistics, asthma attack rates were higher for African Americans and Hispanics. Young children (ages four and under) had the highest rate of hospitalization for asthma, and in 1998, 5,438 people died from asthma. Fragrances also trigger migraines. Women account for about three-quarters of the twenty-eight million adult Americans with migraines. [4] There are many health conditions fragrance exposure can cause and exacerbate.

Less than 1,500 chemicals out of an estimated 5,000 or more fragrance chemicals have been tested for safety by the industry. Multiple chemical sensitivities, allergic reactions, and difficulty breathing are some of the symptoms that 884 toxic substances used in fragrances are capable of causing, according to the National Institute of Occupational Safety and Health. Toluene (methyl benzene) was detected in fragrance samples collected by the EPA in 1991. Toluene is a "hazardous waste." It is flammable and volatile, it attacks the central nervous system, blood, liver, kidneys, eyes, and skin, and it serves as an asthma trigger. The EPA lists Methylene chloride as being among twenty of the most common chemicals in thirty-one tested fragrance products, as a suspected human carcinogen. Methylene chloride is also found in pesticides and septic tank cleaners. Air "fresheners," according to the Household Hazardous Waste Project, do not freshen the air at all. What they do is mask one odor with another, while diminishing one's sense of smell with a nerve-deadening agent. [5]

Synthetic fragrances are capable of causing a number of diseases, many of which a person may not equate to the product. Within this book, you will be able to read some excerpts from scientific journals and opinions from medical experts. I've also included a chemical analysis of a popular perfume, chosen as a big offender by many people.

The fragrance industry is in violation of the Toxic Substances Control Act. Below are some excerpts from the Act.

[Excerpts] Toxic Substances Control Act (TSCA)

The Toxic Substances Control Act of 1976 was enacted by Congress to test, regulate, and screen all chemicals produced or imported into the United States. Many thousands of chemicals and their compounds are developed each year with unknown toxic or dangerous characteristics. To prevent tragic consequences, TSCA requires that any chemical that reaches the consumer marketplace be tested for possible toxic effects prior to commercial manufacture.

Any existing chemical that poses health and environmental hazards is tracked and reported under TSCA. Procedures also are authorized for corrective action under TSCA in cases of cleanup of toxic materials contamination. TSCA supplements other federal statutes, including the Clean Air Act and the Toxic Release Inventory under EPCRA.*

Millions of people are maimed and disabled from repeated exposures to perfume chemicals, and it seems inevitable that there will be millions more. It is estimated that *thirty million* Americans have MCS to varying degrees. [6]

Although MCS is recognized by the Social Security Administration and the Americans with Disabilities Act (ADA) as a legitimate disability, people who suffer from MCS rarely get accommodated anywhere, not even in a medical facility.

There are many other toxic substances in our environment, yet perfumes and other artificially scented products are extremely ubiquitous. They are almost everywhere and virtually impossible to avoid, unless one remains housebound. Even being housebound does not always guarantee safety, as fumes from a neighbor's scented laundry products may waft into an opened window.

There is a very wide range of symptoms caused by fragrances, especially in concealed or confined spaces, including difficulty in breathing and swallowing, asthma, migraines, seizures, fatigue, anaphylaxis (life threatening allergy), short-term memory loss, confusion, disorientation, incoherence, inability to concentrate, nausea, anxiety, irritability, mood swings, irregular heart beats, hypertension, muscle and joint pain, muscle weakness, rashes, hives, eczema, swollen lymph glands, restlessness, flushing, and depression. [7]

It is now documented that different fragrances have different levels of potency and cause different levels of reactions. Researchers at Tulane University in 2001 singled out certain perfumes that triggered asthma worse than others. Out of thirty-eight perfumes, some of them were found to be more potent. For asthmatics, the most potent fragrances were Poison, Opium, Charlie, Red, Giorgio, and White Diamonds. [7]

Many products labeled as *unscented* are oftentimes strongly scented. Some fragrance-free labeled products have been known to contain fragrance chemicals. Hypo-allergenic has no legal meaning.

---

* EPCRA - Emergency Planning and Community Right-to-know Act.

For example, if a child's sunscreen contains fragrance, yet claims to be hypo-allergenic, I would consider this to be an inaccurate statement.

Not everyone experiences the symptoms of exposure to fragrance at the same time, but since fragrances are by definition volatile, they are easily inhaled by others. [7] What may not seemingly bother you today could bother you tomorrow.

HOW PERFUMES HAVE AFFECTED MY LIFE
(My Story)

I had a passion for perfumes and various other fragranced products. Spraying perfume on myself, lathering my hair with fragranced shampoos and conditioners, spreading perfumed lotions on my body, as well as using scented hair gels and lots of hairspray was simply a normal routine before leaving my house every day. Air fresheners and potpourri were used abundantly in my bathrooms and throughout my house. I absolutely loved scented candles. They sure did smell divine.

One morning, out of the blue, my perfume smelled *different* to me. The best word I can use to describe the smell was *stench*. Could this acrid odor be why my boss was usually out of the office? He and I shared a rather small working area. Reminiscing, I could not recall having received many compliments regarding my fragrance of choice. I'd been wearing Confess, the imitation brand of Calvin Klein's Obsession, for quite some time. There is no doubt that I was spraying on more and more perfume in order for me to smell it. I assumed that if I couldn't smell it, no one else could either. Perplexed as I was by this suddenly strange odor, I gave up perfumes, at least the types sprayed from bottles.

From that point on, I could not tolerate being in close proximity to anyone wearing Confess or Obsession. I'd experience an instant, left-sided migraine headache. My left eyelid drooped and heart palpitations often occurred when exposed to the very perfume I had once worn. What was wrong with this perfume? I wondered. Or what was wrong with me? Two of my closest friends (one wore Confess and the other Obsession) now had to refrain from wearing this particular scent while in my presence. At that time, I had no idea that this perfume problem was going to get worse—much worse!

Occasionally, I'd get a whiff of someone's pungent perfume and immediately feel outraged. How *dare* someone wear a fragrance so strong, causing me an instant headache? Perfume exposures would bring out the worst in me. I'd feel hostile and combative. Once out of the person's vapor trail, I would begin to resume normal behavior. The headaches would subside within approximately twenty minutes.

As the years progressed, my headaches became more intense and lasted longer with each perfume exposure. I became quite concerned, as my world started to slowly close in on me. All the while, I was still using certain scented products such as hairspray, body lotions, and air *fresheners,* to name a few.

Shopping at malls or other department stores had become a challenge. I held my breath and ran swiftly past perfume counters. If someone was near me, smelling as if they'd literally bathed in their perfume, I'd become extremely agitated. All in all, though, shopping was something I still enjoyed, although I'd come home quite fatigued.

One Saturday afternoon, my mother, daughter, nephew, and I decided to eat lunch at Round the Corner, a nice hamburger joint located in the mall. Soon after our waitress seated us, a lady, marinated in perfume, was seated in the booth next to ours. Immediately, I stood up and insisted that we be seated as far away from this person as possible. There was no way I could have tolerated any lengthy period of time in close proximity to this woman's perfume.

Several years ago, in the early eighties, I was dining in a Chinese restaurant with my husband. Before finishing our meal, two people were seated in the booth behind us. Their fragrance was extremely overpowering. Both my husband and I could taste it in our food. I glanced over my shoulder, surprised to see two men occupying the booth. I wondered how they could possibly taste their food while so strongly doused in cologne. Prior to the assault, I had been in a pleasant mood, but that quickly changed to anger. Now I often wonder if fragrance chemicals are responsible for so much unexplained hostile behavior.

My oldest daughter used to wear a wretched smelling fragrance in the late-eighties. I checked her room and found a bottle of CK. I remember wondering what was up with *initials* for perfumes. I didn't realize that the initials stood for Calvin Klein at that time. My husband and I insisted she cut down on her usage, as every time she walked past us, we'd nearly suffocate. I remember wondering, what in the world has happened to perfumes? They sure have changed, compared to years past.

If trying to evade perfumes in public places wasn't bad enough, magazines had become scented. A magazine I once subscribed to was now impossible to read, as the scents were overpowering and headache provoking. Far too many magazines are scented these days, so I simply stopped buying them.

More and more perfumes were beginning to bother me. At times, my daughter's friends would stop by wearing perfume, cologne, or aftershave. I insisted that my daughter inform her friends to refrain from wearing scented products within my presence. A few of my own friends began wearing perfumes, and I wanted to avoid being near them. Time and repeated exposures would eventually bring me more misery.

In the 90s, I decided to see a Nutritionist. She suggested I take several capsules, each day, of a *natural* anti-fungal called Candistatin. The Nutritionist thought my adverse reactions to perfumes could possibly be due to a condition called Candida. Not only did I become very sick from taking this supplement but I could have died as a result. I was experiencing severe stomach pains, which lasted for hours at a time. This landed me in the doctor's office. My doctor explained that this supplement might have eventually ruptured my stomach, as it contained alkaloids, which can erode the stomach's lining. The doctor prescribed Prevacid and insisted I be cautious about taking herbal supplements. When I called the Nutritionist to inform her about what had happened to me, she ignored my phone calls.

If not for perfumes bothering me, I never would have tried this remedy in the first place. I continued wondering what could possibly be wrong with me, and why were perfumes causing me so many health problems? How could other people tolerate it? Yet, there had been a time when none of it seemingly bothered *me* either.

Soon enough, scented candles began causing me migraines. It wasn't long before they bothered me even if unlit. I noticed that they seemed to be everywhere—in most gift shops, novelty stores, department stores, grocery stores, and of course, in many people's homes. Is there a safe place to shop? I wondered. Even health food stores sell perfumes, incense, and scented candles.

Many scented body lotions were also causing me to experience headaches. My youngest daughter walked past me one morning, in a rush to leave for work, and I experienced the all too familiar instant "hit." I developed a migraine headache that would make me miserable and irritable. When I confronted my daughter about her perfume use, she adamantly insisted she wasn't *wearing* any. Later, I searched her room and noticed a bottle of body lotion on top of her dresser. The ingredients listed the word "perfume." I threw the bottle away and bought her a fragrance-free lotion. A few friends of mine would occasionally buy me scented lotions for my birthday. I'd immediately discard them into the trashcan. When I first learned the *truth* about perfumes, I went through my entire house—underneath the sinks, linen closet, and laundry room—and threw away every fragranced product I could find. Fragranced products filled my trashcan to the brim. My trash could have easily qualified as a 50-gallon drum of hazardous waste.

Fabric softeners and dryer sheets were also causing me to feel ill. For several years, scented fabric softeners and dryer sheets have been two of my biggest offenders—both on people and spewing into the air from people's dryers. A whiff of the stuff makes my head feel like it's going to explode, and my eyes will burn for hours. If I smell enough of it, I'll start gagging. Petrochemicals, used for laundry purposes, also generate more flammability to clothing.

After a wedding I attended in February of 1999, I knew something in perfumes just had to be very bad. I knew a lot of people didn't like perfumes, but why were they not as sick as me? Three women were heavily scented at this wedding, which prompted me to leave the reception much earlier than I had initially planned.

It was obvious that my reactions to fragrances were continuing to worsen, and it took less exposure to incapacitate me. My left eye began to ache, along with the drooping eyelid, and at times, I'd feel sharp pains in my left eye. I could feel a sore "knot" in my left temple and was experiencing *new* symptoms, such as burning nostrils, dizziness, loss of balance, more *frequent* heart palpitations, extreme fatigue, muscle aches, depression, episodes of gagging, and occasionally dry heaves upon some exposures. The headaches were becoming more intense and lasting longer, sometimes for days. This is not a normal migraine, in my opinion. After the Tylenol wore off, I'd wake up the next morning with a perfume hangover. It is a very sick feeling involving head pain, burning eyes, nausea, and weakness. Unless you suffer from these reactions, you can only imagine.

Every single outing had become a crapshoot, as man-made fragrances are ubiquitous. It's nearly impossible to enter a building without encountering perfume chemicals. Fragrance chemicals are also quite abundant outdoors as well.

Walking through grocery store aisles, where detergents, soaps, cleaning products, shampoos, and conditioners are sold, began causing me disconcerting symptoms. Entering a friend's home, which I used to enter without any trepidation, had become risky. Weddings, baby showers, and most social gatherings became events I must now avoid. Receiving an invitation to any get-together is anxiety provoking, as I must decline again and again, with the exception of a few friends who are willing to accommodate me as best they can.

Fragrance chemicals often alienate people from each other. To say this is sad is an understatement. How was I going to live the rest of my life as a primarily housebound person? How would this affect my relationships with my husband, daughters, and my friends? I'm still relatively young, so what is one to do? It took lower levels of exposures to debilitate me, even if outdoors. My husband, mother, daughters, and friends have become "sniffing guide people" for me. This is no way to live, yet I'd soon learn that *millions* of Americans live this way.

How can a country that touts the importance of education permit this atrocity? Millions of people are inhaling neurotoxic chemicals every day. What about freedom? There are millions of people who are virtually prisoners of their homes due to ubiquitous fragrance chemicals, and the numbers continue to grow.

By April of 1999, I'd become primarily housebound. Going to the doctor usually makes me ill. I presented my doctor with Anderson Laboratories, Inc. scientific journal, Acute Toxic Effects of Fragrance Products, and he made a copy for himself. He said it appeared to him as though my central nervous system was adversely affected by perfumes. I delayed much needed dental work for nearly two years. Many people, I'd learn, do not visit a doctor or dentist at all, and their biggest fear is the possibility of going to a hospital. They would rather die at home then go to a facility, which exists for the sole purpose of *health,* due to fragrance exposures. Nearly every outing brings physical suffering, and yet I'd believe that there *must* be a cure for this affliction.

Perplexed by my illness, I searched the Internet for answers. I joined a Listserv group by the name of Fragranced Products Information Network (FPIN) headed by Betty Bridges, RN. This group was strictly for activists—people trying to spread the word and educate others about the dangers of fragranced products. This was the first time I'd actually *see* the ingredients in these products that were making me sick. It was absolutely mortifying, to say the least. Prior to joining the group, I had been hoping to find a remedy, antidote, or possibly a cure.

What I learned is not pretty. Many of the chemicals in perfumes, and other artificially scented products, are listed on the EPA's Hazardous Waste List.[1] Hardly fresh, clean, pure, healthy, or alluring.

This newfound knowledge led me to embark on a new journey—over four years of activism, thus far. All the while, there have been countless others who have preceded me, working towards the same cause. Some people have been working for decades, trying to bring forth awareness regarding this chemical cover-up. People have tried diligently to generate some much needed and long overdue laws, so people who experience life-threatening reactions to fragrance chemicals can receive accommodation. I suppose that until there are laws banning fragrance use in public buildings, accommodation would be difficult to enforce. If people are suddenly asked to refrain from wearing scented products, they are going to ask questions. Long kept *secrets* could be revealed.

Through the FPIN Listserv group, I corresponded with many intelligent and dedicated people. Betty Bridges has compiled incredible in-depth information regarding synthetic fragrances, available on her website. I also corresponded with Barb Wilke, current President of the Environmental Health Network of California. She is a major activist and also has an in-depth website of her own. These two women have devoted many years to their research, much of which has been obtained *from* the perfume industries.

I met quite a few interesting people in this group. There are countless people working towards the same cause, yet we still have no guaranteed accommodation. I was not at all pleased by what I learned. I was stunned!

The first article I read regarding the contents in fabric softeners and dryer sheets was enough to repulse me, and many of these chemicals are also abundant in perfumes. What I found shocking is that many fragrance chemicals are not even *meant* to be inhaled or touched, yet they are being sold specifically for that very purpose. Many fragrance chemicals do not have Material Safety Data Sheets (MSDS) listed for them, which is required by law. The more I learned, the more determined I became to spread the word.

During my involvement with the FPIN group, I met Hollie. She shared her personal misfortune with me, in regards to perfumes. She was also a *former* user. In fact, she had once owned over one hundred bottles of the stuff. Hollie told me she was in a movie theater, several years ago, when a lady sat near her, drenched in Giorgio perfume. The perfume caused Hollie to projectile vomit. After twenty-three years of working as a legal secretary, Hollie is disabled from repeated exposures to perfumes.

I heard about a monthly publication called *Our Toxic Times*, Chemical Injury Information Network (CIIN), founded by Cynthia Wilson, in 1990. Shortly thereafter, I heard of yet another newsletter, *The N.O.S.E.* (The Northern Ohio Sensitivity Extra). I subscribed to both of these publications for a while. This is simply more validation of how rampant MCS has become. I had never heard of the term multiple chemical sensitivities until the year 1999, although I certainly have had it for a long time.

I wrote letters to several major hospitals within the Denver Metro Area explaining the dangers of fragranced products. It seemed logical to me that they might take an interest, considering their sole purpose of existence is for promoting health. One person from The Children's Hospital in Denver called me at home, apparently interested in the information. I spoke with people affiliated with the National Jewish Hospital in Denver. They do their best to implement a fragrance-free environment for their asthma patients, along with a fragrance-free adjoining school.

It's very sad to discover that many children cannot tolerate living in civilization due to perfume exposures causing them life-threatening asthma attacks. Why doesn't the National Jewish Hospital get more involved with this issue? I wondered. Could it be because they are government funded? This seems to be the case with many health care facilities. I'd also learn that many government entities—such as the Environmental Protection Agency (EPA), the Consumer Product Safety Commission (CPSC), the Department of Health, the Federal Trade Commission (FTC), Occupational Safety & Health Administration (OSHA), Agency for Toxic Substance and Disease Registry (ATSDR), Comprehensive Environmental Response, Compensation, and Liability Act of 1980 (CERCLA), the Department of Justice, and the Center for Disease Control (CDC)—were of very little help when it came to the subject of perfumes.

After writing to various health groups, Internet newsgroups, politicians, and newspapers, my efforts seemed futile. I called churches, restaurant owners, anyone who would listen, but my efforts continued to fall upon deaf ears. Contacting HMOs seemed like a good idea. Hollie and I sent packets of information in the mail to several HMO Chief Executive Officers. Neither she nor I heard a word back from any of them.

I contacted several HMOs via email recently and received quite a few positive responses thanking me for the information. It seems to boil down to money—who's making it and who's losing it. Recently, I've heard from several people informing me that many churches are asking their parishioners to ease up on their perfumes and other scented products, although not asking them to completely refrain. This certainly is not happening because of anything *I've* done but because perfumes really do bother millions of people throughout the entire country. Actually, it's a global problem. I understand people simply wanting to smell nice, but at the expense of being toxic, is it worth it? I think not.

Important steps in the right direction began to unfold…

The Environmental Health Network of California filed a petition with the FDA, in May of 1999, requesting the Commissioner to take administrative action and declare "Eternity" eau de parfum by Calvin Klein Cosmetic Company, misbranded. Eternity was chosen because many peopled cited it as a big offender. This doesn't mean other perfumes or fragrances are any safer, by any means. The responses that were flooding in from medical experts were phenomenal. This seemed promising, yet presently, the petition is still open for comments.

In July of 1999, an article appeared in the *Wall Street Journal.* Halifax, Nova Scotia had implemented a fragrance-free policy. Before a substitute teacher could return to work, she had been instructed to go home and shower off her perfume. People in hospitals were ordered to towel down if too heavily scented. Besides public institutions, many private businesses ask people to refrain from using perfumes or scents. This is the fragrance industry's worst nightmare coming true, and the trend is spreading in Canada. Fragrance-free is now the policy at a high school outside of Toronto. Public buses request riders to be scent-free in Ottawa. What happened to cause this scenic port city to be the first to set such a trend? Could it be that Canadians care more about their people than the U.S., for example? Hundreds of Camp Hill Medical Centre staff members became ill in 1991 after the hospital's kitchen dishwasher fumes were sucked into the ventilation system. To this day, many of the hundreds of workers remain ill, although the system has been repaired. In most of Halifax, the *norm* is fragrance-free. Violators must go home and shower, without pay. [8]

Talking to a few lawyers, armed with an abundance of evidence, might generate a class-action lawsuit, hopefully bringing forth *awareness*, which is desperately needed. The deception *must* be stopped. There are certainly countless potential plaintiffs.

I've talked with strangers who claim that their wife's spray of perfume in the morning is the worst part of their day. One lady told me that she and her husband sleep in separate bedrooms because they can't stand each other's fragrance. I know people who are bothered by their *own* perfume, so they dab a "little" on their ankles or the back of their neck. Is this insane or what? Never in my life had I thought of suing anyone or any company, but this industry *deserves* to get sued for the damage it's caused to the health of millions of people, for their deception, for their product's liability, and for their failure to bear warning labels. If you think you're not being affected, are your health insurance premiums skyrocketing?

The first lawyer I spoke to suggested that I move to a small city. I told her that I couldn't simply pack my belongings and move, nor should I have to, and what about the millions of others? What kind of justice would that be? Her suggestion was the best she could offer.

I started collecting various newspaper and online articles pertaining to fragranced products. One morning, I spotted a brief article about illnesses caused by an air freshener. A can of solid air freshener, which had been left in an elevator, overheated and erupted. Thirty-two people became sick in the post's Army Community Services building, experiencing nausea, vomiting, headaches, and burning eyes, and were sent to Evans Army Hospital, where they were treated and released. After two days of detective work, the solid air freshener was found. It had overheated while next to the elevator's mechanical systems, allowing toxic fumes to enter the building. [25]

Wearing cologne caused three seventh-graders to be suspended from school for three days. A teacher, Jean Bartlett, at Cedarcrest Middle School is sensitive to scented products. Although the boys had been informed of Bartlett's sensitivities by their regular teacher, and signs were posted in Bartlett's class reminding students of her severe allergies, the boys admitted to wearing the cologne in order to get excused from class. The manager of community relations for the school district, Mary Fears, commented that they had honored Jean Bartlett's disability. Respiratory arrest could have occurred. But one parent thought this suspension was not fair and suggested Ms. Bartlett work at an Elementary school where fragrances are not as abundant. The boys' suspension was later reduced to one day. The possible grave circumstances were something the boys, more than likely, didn't fully understand. [26]

These incidents are actually very common . . .

In the summer of 2000, a lawyer gave us false hope. He asked us to present him with ten potential plaintiffs, all from one state, which we did. We had more than ten, but provided him with at least ten from California. California seemed like a good place to start, due to Proposition 65, which requires the governor to publish a list of chemicals that are known to the state of California to cause cancer, birth defects, or other reproductive harm. This list must be updated at least once a year. Over 700 chemicals have been added as of March 10, 2000. After the lawyer discussed our "hopeful" case with a sister law firm, we were declined.

I read the potential plaintiff's letters, and they were all heartbreaking. One lady, who had never used perfumes or fragrances, acquired MCS due to the use of her co-worker's perfumes; therefore, she retired from her job early. Another lady was so sensitive and ill from repeated exposures to fragrance products that she became housebound and was unable to attend her own son's wedding. One lady mentioned that her thirteen-year old son could not attend public schools, as he experiences a reduction in breathing from perfumes. He has had this medical condition for ten years. Another lady was approved for Social Security Disability because of her sensitivity to fragrance. She has a B.S. degree in business administration, so she obviously would rather be *able* to work. Her condition (MCS) was confirmed by MDs, neurologists, psychologists, psychiatrists, and anesthesiologists. A lady, whose sixteen-year old son has had MCS since the age of seven, tried to get accommodation for him at school, unsuccessfully. His teacher told his mother that she was bothered by fragrances, too, yet feared losing her job should she complain. Another lady, an RN, developed MCS in 1994. It happened quite suddenly for her, and she is now a prisoner of her home. After twenty-five years of dedicated service in hospital work, she is now reclusive and disabled. She was one of many who mentioned how exposures to fragrances caused her to feel not only sick but also combative.

All the potential plaintiffs have trouble with social gatherings, shopping, and simple tasks, as perfumes are everywhere. How very much I could relate to these sad and true stories. The stories I read were from people who suffered tremendously, yet they are only a minute fraction of the people who suffer from synthetic fragrances. Millions of lives are forever changed.

I pursued another lawyer, who reminded me of my statute of limitations. I have long surpassed my statute of limitations, which is two years in Colorado. How could I have *known* that I was chemically injured by perfumes, when several years were spent wondering *why* perfumes and colognes made me so sick? The fact that I felt well *until* exposed to perfumes was a mystery to me. I thought that hazardous products were labeled as such. I soon realized that the possibility of judicial corruption is too high, which was probably the reason for this enormous lack of justice. Suddenly, the situation seemed clear to me. The idea of continuing a search for a lawyer, whether toxic tort, consumer fraud, or environmental law, would probably be a waste of my time.

Not surprisingly, one lawyer shared that his own wife has MCS and is intolerant of perfumes, and another said that walking past perfume counters caused him to feel nauseated.

Once a person acquires MCS, life becomes quite challenging. Simple pleasures, once taken for granted, are no longer the same. For example, something as simple as a barbecue with friends could become a physically sickening experience—or possibly life-threatening. Running to the grocery store when out of a few items isn't worth the risk. Having unexpected company may cause illness, if they are scented. Sometimes, even my own family members forget to refrain from using scented personal care products, such as fragranced hair gel or a scented deodorant. It's difficult when so few products are fragrance-free.

What I find alarming is how quickly this permanent injury can occur and how many people currently *have* this affliction. Many people who wear perfume often tell me that scented candles give them instant headaches. Many people can't stand someone else's perfume, yet assume their own is acceptable. What these people do not realize is that this is how MCS begins for many of us. For some people, MCS may be preceded by an exposure to another toxic substance, such as pesticides, formaldehyde out-gassing from new carpets, or exposures to an herbicide or insecticide for a few examples. Usually, though, it is the ubiquitous fragrance chemicals that keep most chemically injured people sick, housebound, and isolated. For me, it was undoubtedly my own perfume that starting the ball rolling. I *know* it, but how could I ever prove it? Unfortunately, many people will probably continue using their hazardous substances until it makes *them* sick.

I contacted the owner of my favorite Mexican restaurant. Usually I could dine there with minimal exposures, but a new waitress had been hired. She polluted the small restaurant all by herself. The owner called me, thanking me for my letter, yet said she would not request any of her waitresses to refrain from wearing their perfumes. She further explained that it was her "religion" to wear perfume. Not long ago, my daughter ate lunch there and told me that the restaurant is now burning incense inside the non-smoking establishment. She could taste the chemicals in her food. My desire to dine at that restaurant again is history. I'd rather smell the aroma of food instead of hazardous waste chemicals. It's not the *smell* that's sickening but the chemicals.

My brother worked at a warehouse in northern Denver where there are open, empty fields. He told me about one Hispanic co-worker who wore a ton of cologne. Not only did the rabbits and other wildlife, which once frequented the area, disappear after this man came on board but the cologne wearer himself was consistently calling in sick. Wildlife animals seem to have an intuition when it comes to danger. My brother is not chemically sensitive, yet claimed that this one man's cologne gave *him* a headache.

My friend Mary complained that she had been experiencing an unrelenting headache for weeks on end, without any let up. She visited several doctors, yet not one doctor could figure out what might be the culprit. I asked her if she had scented candles in her house and she answered, saying that nearly every room in her house had one burning. After removing the scented candles from her home, Mary's prolonged headache eventually subsided and has not returned. Honestly, doctors need to be asking the same questions when their patients complain of unexplained headaches, as not everyone readily equates their health ailments to the source. Doctors should also be warning people to avoid fragrances if they have asthma, and certainly oncologists should be warning their cancer patients of the risks involved, as well as neurologists. The fragrance industry, I'd imagine, certainly keeps pharmaceutical companies, neurologists, oncologists, and doctors who treat asthma and chronic migraines in big business.

Curious, I decided to interview several high school students, who were friends of my youngest daughter. I was not surprised to learn that many of them admitted suffering *daily* headaches from classmates' perfumes and other scented products. Little do they know, they may become *more* sensitized with time and repeated exposures.

It only takes one heavily scented person to engulf an entire room, leaving behind a vapor trail lingering in the air for a very long time. Have you ever noticed that some people's fragrance is so notably strong that you can taste it in your mouth? Or have you noticed that some people's fragrance can be smelled, even if eighty feet away from you? A lady I once worked with, long ago, used to douse herself in perfume. Her odor was still in the office by Monday morning, although she had been away since the prior Friday evening.

Co-workers frequently commented that they could smell where she'd been. Sometimes, men use strongly scented deodorants or aftershave, smelling as if they'd poured an entire bottle of cologne over their head. There are numerous occasions when one person will pollute the air in an entire store, restaurant, or any building for that matter. And we wonder what's wrong with people these days. Almost everyone in this country is being bombarded with a barrage of hazardous chemicals on a daily basis.

Fortunately, I have a husband who works and who has not abandoned me, as so many do. Often, wives leave husbands who have this illness. Some people with MCS do not have spouses and end up losing their careers, homes, and oftentimes their friends. If they are not granted disability, many people end up living with a family member or friends, if feasible. Some people simply become homeless.

Both *Extra* and *Inside Edition* aired a segment about MCS sometime around the end of 1999. The story was about a young lady named Julie, from Evergreen, Colorado. She was a flight attendant for United Airlines. After boarding an airplane that had been sprayed with pesticides, she suffered immediate, life-threatening reactions, which ruined her immune system. She is one of the people now living in the deserts of Arizona with nothing more than a tent, her dog, two horses, and somehow she managed to get water and a phone line. She said fragrances bother her so much that one whiff of someone's scent makes her physically ill. Her voice sounded very raspy, and she looked tired and worn out. Her doctor conducted tests and confirmed that her condition is very real, but the American Medical Association (AMA) does not recognize MCS, which was her diagnosis, as a legitimate illness. This could have much to do with mainstream doctors' ties with pharmaceutical industries, or it may simply be ignorance. For some people, it can be one unfortunate exposure to a toxic substance. I believe this could happen to anyone.

One Congresswoman, Janice Schakowsky, (D) ILL, introduced the Bill HR 1947—Safe Notification Information for Fragrances Act (SNIFF)—on May 22, 2001, to amend the Federal Food, Drug, and Cosmetic Act to require that fragrances containing known toxic substances or allergens be labeled accordingly. This was Janice Schakowsky's second attempt. I applaud her efforts, but there were only two co-sponsors. [9]

It's been difficult explaining to friends why I cannot go many places with them anymore—places I once went without any trouble. Fortunately, many friends have stayed in touch with me, but there are some who may think my condition is possibly contagious, as I can account for a few friends I haven't heard from within the last three to four years. How much fun can a person be when they can't really go to many places? Putting friends aside, it's far more difficult to miss out on important family functions, such as seeing my granddaughter ride a pony at Heritage Square for the first time. Before my youngest daughter turned twenty-one, I had promised to take her to Blackhawk, which is a casino town in Colorado. By the time she turned twenty-one, it was already too late for me. Never would I have dreamed that my life would be reduced to such isolation due to fragrances. Fragrance chemicals are the only thing keeping me from having a normal social life.

My oldest daughter boards a plane to visit us, yearly. Instead of shopping together, as we used to, she offered to grocery shop for me. I gave her my driver's license and a signed check so she could fill in the dollar amount. She explained to the cashier that she was shopping for a "shut-in." Can't say I really liked the *label,* but it happened to be true. For the most part, I *was* and still *am* a "shut-in."

Knowing that my illness began with the daily use of my chosen perfume infuriates me. I had a *right* to know that I was slowly poisoning myself. For many people, it's often second-hand exposures from other people's fragrances that may cause their illness. After days or weeks of being inside my house, I occasionally decide to venture out, as it does the soul good. Rarely do I have a successful outing.

Camping, once or twice, in the summer months is something I still look forward to. Yet, fragrance chemicals are not even escapable in the fresh, crisp air of the mountains. Some people bring along their scented sunscreens, and oftentimes people's clothing will reek of strongly scented laundry chemicals. I supply fragrance-free products for everyone to use, and my friends are careful about their chemical use when in my company.

I've attempted a couple of trips to the Denver Zoo. The fragrance chemicals were very abundant, even outdoors. I had to hold numerous tissues over my nose and mouth. I went to the zoo so that my granddaughter would have some memories of me, besides being at home most of the time.

According to a report in a recent issue of the journal, *Allergy,* irritants can be absorbed via the eyes. Dr. Eva. Millquist and colleagues from the University of Gothenburg reported that after inhaling perfume, people exhibited shortness of breath and also developed a cough. During thirty minutes of exposure to perfume, it was found that there was a gradual increase in eye irritation, shortness of breath, and cough, whether by eyes or airway. This reaction was not seen upon subjects that were exposed to a placebo. [10]

Richard H. Conrad, Ph.D. and Biochemist, told me that a *damp* cloth will help better than the tissues, and recently, I've heard the same suggestion on the news when people are attempting to go outside while the air is blowing smoke our way from wildfires. But he also suggested wearing a Wilson Mask made from Lab Safety Supply. What kind of a toxic country *is* this? We'd probably *all* be wise to wear a Wilson Mask. Wiser yet, would be to stop buying and using toxic products. Ironically, some people with MCS have worn masks, only to be questioned by police as to why.

My husband has attended four weddings, without me, since I've had full-blown MCS. I used to love attending weddings, but weddings or going to church is when people are more apt to spray their scents on awfully thick. Personally, I don't feel like dressing-up in my nicest apparel only to cover my face with a VOC mask. There are so many events I've missed, and there will undoubtedly be more. The inability to avoid scented people makes life challenging and difficult once you've lost your tolerance to these potent and powerful hazardous chemicals.

Certain events I felt I *couldn't* miss, such as my granddaughter's second birthday party at a Chuck E. Cheese, brought me a miserable migraine. Many tears have been shed over these kinds of situations. Many dreams have been lost. Planning an exciting vacation, or flying in an airplane, are just memories now.

Why is it that approximately thirty million or more Americans can detect smells, much like that of a Bloodhound? A dear friend of mine had breast cancer. She told me that after her chemotherapy treatments, her sense of smell was significantly heightened. People with MCS generally acquire a heightened sense of smell. Is this a sign of a compromised immune system? We need more answers. Why doesn't *everyone* have perfume chemical intolerance? Millions of people already do, including people from other countries. We didn't all get to this point at the exact same time. Also, drugs can affect people differently. One person may have some other incurable disease, such as cancer, life-threatening asthma, multiple sclerosis, or one of the many other neurological diseases that scented products may cause. Politicians and celebrities *also* succumb to multiple sclerosis and other neurological and central nervous system diseases, and they are not immune to cancer, either. Fragrance chemicals could possibly be one of the causes of mysterious crib deaths.

A few years ago, during a mammogram procedure, the technician was heavily doused in perfume. I was sick with a migraine the remainder of the day. Ironic, considering perfumes may cause breast cancer. [12] My gynecologist is an intelligent woman, and she has a sign at the reception desk requesting patients and visitors to refrain from wearing scented products due to their chemically sensitive patients *and* staff. Still, I must walk through a maze of toxins in order to get inside her office, since it's located on the third floor. It would be nice to see more doctors and dentists implementing this protocol. She has all her patients sign a piece of paper stating they will refrain from wearing fragrances while in her medical quarters. Twenty-five or thirty years ago, this would have been almost unheard of, but people sickened by fragrances have become quite the epidemic. I think the toxicity is catching up with people at an alarmingly fast pace. In fact, during the beginning of my illness, I felt somewhat stigmatized. Today, there are millions of us, and it seems most people know of someone else, besides themselves, who has this *problem* to some degree.

Many people have tried just about everything imaginable for a cure, from sauna detoxifications, to colon cleanses, coffee enemas, and acupuncture. Many have invested thousands of dollars for the help of alternative and environmental doctors. I have had numerous acupuncture treatments, yet as of this writing, I'm still severely chemically sensitive to perfumes. Unfortunately, most people with MCS or E.I. (Environmental Illness) cannot afford such expensive doctors or treatments. Nor do alternative treatments work for everyone.

I adhered to the Candida diet while taking prescription anti-fungal medications, in hopes that it might lessen my severe symptoms to perfume exposures. I was very faithful to the no sugar, bread, white flour, pasta, white rice, moldy foods, such as cheese and peanuts, and no vinegar diet. I lost a lot of weight, but my chemical sensitivities did *not* improve.

Cutting my own hair has become easier with practice. Eventually, I found a beautician who doesn't wear perfume, and she was willing to use my own products. I bring protection, as well, due to the scented *goods* inside the salon.

When I think of the money I'm *not* spending on frequent professional haircuts, it adds up. It sums up, big time, when I think of the money I cannot spend on airline tickets, hotels, accessories for my home, concerts, movie theater tickets, etc. I purchase less clothing, dine out less, and avoid most shopping centers, especially stores with perfume counters. Do you think this does *not* affect our economy? It most certainly does.

I've discovered many people, *locally,* have the same illness. One of them has been a friend of mine for many years. Perfumes cause her to experience headaches, burning eyes, fatigue, and recently, she told me that perfumes are now causing her to experience chest pains. My next door neighbor's daughter is also sensitive to perfumes. One of her co-workers used a desk fan, deliberately, to waft the scents of potpourri her way. He was fired from his job for having done so.

In time, I heard about a support group for people with *my* problem. Of course, this support group has never been advertised in the newspapers, like so many other support groups are. Gee, I can't imagine why. Could it be the extremely expensive and constant full, one-page fragrance ads? This group, The Rocky Mountain Environmental Health Association (RMEHA), acquainted me with even *more* people who have this affliction.

A little magazine, *AWAKE,* was passed around in my neighborhood the summer of 2000. The magazine mentioned MCS as a growing problem in the U.S. One lady who suffers from MCS said that certain chemicals make her feel drugged, and she'd experience an array of symptoms, ranging from personality changes, to depression, lethargy, and agitation, and her reactions would last anywhere from hours to several days. She mentioned the hung-over feeling that so many people with MCS know only too well. Dr. Claudia Miller commented that these effects are not unusual for people with MCS. She also stated that people exposed often to **solvents** are at a higher risk of developing depression and panic attacks. More frightening, she added, chemical exposures to the brain might be the most sensitive of organ system. The book, *Chemical Exposures – Low Levels and High Stakes,* claims that solvents are among the leading cause of patients who suffer from MCS. Side effects from chemicals can be serious, resulting in death. Some of the side effects, besides shortness of breath and panic attack, are heart palpitations, increased pulse rate, and fluid buildup in the lungs. Symptoms can vary from person to person and include headaches, muscle and joint pain, asthma, sinus problems, anxiety, depression, insomnia, difficulty concentrating, memory problems, irregular heartbeats, fatigue, intestinal problems, nausea, vomiting, and seizures. [11]

The more people I correspond with, the more people they talk to. A friend of my mother, after hearing about my perfume intolerance, shared that her *own* mother wouldn't leave her house, the last five years of her life, because perfumes made her extremely ill. This elderly lady did not own a computer, nor did she have awareness or knowledge regarding the harmful effects of perfumes. I spoke to an elderly lady whom I met through the Rocky Mountain Environmental Health Association. She was concerned about us *younger* people with perfume intolerance. Perfumes make her very sick. She was a former user of various fragrant products, much like me. She stated that most of her friends, who wore perfumes, were already dead of something or another. Sure, it could simply be coincidence, but her statement was candid.

There have been a few times I've thought of driving to Halifax, Nova Scotia. It would be nice to have a few safe places to go without the constant assaults from perfumes. I studied the Atlas one evening to see exactly how to make the drive. Of course, this is an unrealistic dream for me, as I have family here. But it's still a dream that is always on my mind. Living like a prisoner, when I didn't commit a crime, is a nightmare. When I was growing up, I never would have dreamed that perfumes, of all things, would ruin my life. I am undoubtedly not alone. It would be nice to have a little freedom, justice, and accommodation, especially in a doctor's office, of all places.

Even a drive-thru restaurant doesn't guarantee escape from exposures. Often, the person at the window may reek of perfume, and the breeze swiftly brings it into my car. I've dropped mail off in drive-thru mailboxes at the post office, and the stench from the person in the car before me was still lingering in a pocket of air. It's ridiculous. It doesn't seem to matter where I might venture. If there is one person doused in perfume, they often end up standing or sitting right next to me. Have I become a perfume magnet? There honestly doesn't seem to be *any* public building free of the toxic chemical stew.

Three years ago, I called a local grocery store inquiring into home delivery. The gentleman I spoke to stated that although there are various reasons for home delivery, perfume intolerance is a growing problem and reason for home delivery. Home delivery is not cheap either.

My friend, Janine, missed out on a long-time planned vacation with her husband and two children due to her inability to tolerate fragrance chemicals. Janine stayed home for ten days, while her husband and children went to Disney Land. She also missed out on a long-time planned trip to Hawaii with her parents. Their trip to Hawaii had been planned for the year 1999, but by 1998, Janine was already too sick.

Difficult for many, since acquiring MCS, is the inability to help others. How can we help a person in need of medical attention when we cannot even tolerate the fragrance chemicals in the hospital, for instance? Should a person who is wearing a strong scent need CPR, they'd better hope I'm not the only person around. I'm the kind of person who would try to help, but I could end up passing out or getting too sick before being able to complete the technique. I had a very difficult time accompanying my daughter while her own daughter was sick. The health care facility had receptionists who reeked of their chemical cocktails.

People should be concerned about where these toxic chemicals may end up. Get a whiff of this. In Leon, Mexico, a perfume-factory manager and several employees spread *eight tons* of perfume on one of Mexico City's main freeways. This was done so citizens could "smell" the impending change in Mexico's government. This bizarre stunt caused eighteen cars to skid out of control, sustaining damage, as well as a temporary shutdown of a major artery. [27]

I can only *imagine* what may have happened had someone lit a match. What will happen in the future to their underground water supply? This stunt was simply careless and reckless on behalf of the perfume industry.

The summer of 2001, my husband and I went to Thermopolis, Wyoming for a brief, much needed getaway. Even in Wyoming, fragrance chemicals cannot be avoided. I do have to admit, less people tend to wear fragrances in smaller cities, but it's abundant in public restrooms and gift shops. When I entered a gift shop and got a whiff of the polluting scented candles, I exited immediately. We were very fortunate to "luck out" in most of the restaurants, though. How refreshing it was to enjoy a meal without breathing toxic fumes for a change. Thermopolis, Wyoming is not exactly my vision of a dream vacation of a lifetime, but it is a great city. It was very relaxing to get away from the big city life, and our motel managers accommodated me very nicely.

When I'm not breathing fragrance chemicals, for a few days, my energy level increases, and my mood is calm. The lines under my eyes diminish, and I feel more alive. But a person *must* get out, now and then, although, for millions of us, certainly not very often.

Not long ago, I decided to sport a designer charcoal filtered mask. It's a mask, which is made to look somewhat tasteful, if you can imagine. I have two of them. My friend, Terri, wore my spare mask so I wouldn't feel singled out. Not having been to a mall in a very long time, I thought I'd try it. We looked like a couple of bandits, or possibly members of a new gang of some kind. People not only stared at us, they ran directly up to us, asking, "Why the masks?"

I'm grateful to have met Terri, as she is very considerate of my perfume sensitivities and not too many people I know, personally, will don a mask for a friend. Even with the mask, I felt as if I was suffocating, and it didn't filter out enough of the chemicals. It was better than no protection at all, but I *did* end up sick.

In May of 2002, my husband's mother passed away. Her funeral was in Bessemer, PA. I should have been able to be by my husband's side in his time of grief. I knew there was no way my health would allow it, as perfumes are in the airport, airplane, and in people's homes. Many homes are filled with scented soaps, detergents, fabric softeners, and scented candles, which *are* perfumes. I stayed home.

While reading a world briefing in the newspaper, I spotted yet another article. Nineteen people in Saudi Arabia died from drinking cologne, and seventeen people were hospitalized. The cologne happened to contain methanol, which is a poisonous substance often used in antifreeze. Since drinking alcohol in Saudi Arabia is not permitted, unless one wants to endure lashings, some people drink cologne as an alcohol substitute. [28]

Slowly but surely, news is spreading. *The New York Times,* July 11, 2002, pg. A17, contained a full, one-page ad with a picture of a pregnant woman holding a bottle of perfume up to her nose. The ad stressed the dangers of phthalates—how toxic and poisonous these chemicals can be to the unborn. Damage to the lungs, kidneys, liver, and the developing testes of the fetus can result from the use of phthalates. The ad was sponsored by Coming Clean, the Environmental Working Group and Health Care Without Harm.

A woman in Florida was arrested for spraying herself with perfume, burning scented candles, and using bug killer and disinfectant in an attempt to seriously injure her husband, David Taylor. The incident occurred on April 4, 2003. David was exposed to toxic mold and hazardous chemicals while employed as a construction worker, which triggered his chemical sensitivities. Investigators were provided with a letter from Taylor's physician confirming that he suffers from sensitivity to volatile chemicals, including all fragrances and air fresheners, and that his wife is aware of it. Lynda Taylor was charged with aggravated battery.[29] David's story has been shared in *People Magazine* and also aired on *Good Morning America, Inside Edition,* and *CNN*.

Could perfumes and other artificially scented products be why there are so many diseases with unknown causes and no cures? Could these products be why so many more children are now getting leukemia and various other cancers, or why more women are diagnosed with breast cancer, and at younger ages? Could this be why neurological diseases are on the rise, and Multiple Sclerosis, chemical sensitivities, and asthma have increased to epidemic proportions?

Please do not be fooled by deceptive advertising. Fragrances are not healthy products, and I wouldn't suggest poisoning the people who raised you by purchasing fragrances on Mother's Day or Father's Day. The same goes for Valentine's Day, and of course, the biggest shopping holiday of the year, Christmas. The fragrance industry advocates their advertisements, abundantly, before all of these holidays. There is *not,* in my opinion, a good time to buy *anyone* these products. People could be creative and buy the special people in their lives gifts such as musical CDs, movies, picture frames, gift certificates for dinner at their favorite restaurant, or any number of other gift ideas for that matter.

Having been a very sociable person most of my life, I must now *avoid* people. I miss my freedom. Fragrance chemicals have ruined my life, as I once knew it, and the lives of millions of people.

Had I *known* about the toxicity of perfumes and other scented products, I would have chosen not to use them, and I would have stayed clear of people who did.

I continue to live with MCS and spend the majority of my time at home.

CHAPTER 1

PERFUMES AND THE CANCER CONNECTION

CONNIE PITTS

GET A WHIFF OF THIS

CANCER RESEARCH CENTER OF AMERICA, INC.

Dr. James W. Coleman
President/CEO of Cancer Research Center of America, Inc.

The following is a summary from Dr. Coleman's work.

Cosmetics Linked to the Causes of Breast Cancer and Fatal Breast Cancer

Medical Overview
About 180,000 women in the United States will develop breast cancer each year and 43,500 women will die, annually, from this disease. *All* women are at risk. To better understand this topic, some basic medical facts would be helpful. These statistics are alarming considering breast cancer is essentially a preventable disease, even among women with a genetic predisposition.

How breast cancer can develop may be helpful in understanding why this is essentially a preventable disease. A breast contains millions of cells. Cancer could develop with any one of these cells located beneath the skin. A normal breast cell does not become cancerous spontaneously but may become cancerous only after it has been exposed to either a chemical agent or ionizing radiation that is capable of damaging DNA or causing the cell to mutate. To become cancerous, the DNA must mutate or become damaged twice in the same region of the same cell. This damage or mutation occurs after a normal breast cell has been repeatedly exposed to a carcinogenic agent, depending on the particular agent, for a period of five to forty years.

Regulating and Testing
The *only* agency mandated by Congress to regulate cosmetics—the Cosmetics Act of 1938—is the U.S. Food and Drug Administration (FDA). Yet, the FDA has no authority to prohibit a cosmetic manufacturer from using certain carcinogenic ingredients in

producing their products. Fragrances, toiletries, and other personal care products are *not* covered under the **Act**, as they are *not* classified as cosmetics.

The FDA conducts a limited amount of testing, even with cosmetics, due to budgetary constraints. If a carcinogen is found, enforcement by this agency is unlikely. The general public mistakenly believes that cosmetics containing carcinogens are not marketed.

Many **mainstream** advocates of breast health boast that before marketing, many beauty aids and cosmetics are testing "rigorously." They do not inform the public that testing is done by the manufacturers. Manufacturers mainly test for immediate allergic reactions, irritation to skin, and flammability of aerosol products. Published evidence of any product study with humans, by the manufacturers, for injuries resulting from carcinogens that may develop after five to fifteen years of exposure is not known.

Breast health advocates who make deceptive statements regarding "rigorous" testing generally have financial ties to one or more of the offending industries. Persons from these industries have infiltrated and become entrenched in the FDA and some *mainstream* breast health organizations.

Some editors of **medical journals** have ties to one or more of the offending industries. As a result, the general public may cast light favorably to the offending industries, due to biased information.

Occupational Connection

Female beauticians, cosmetologists, and hairdressers handle hair dyes and organic solvents in many nail care products, hair sprays, and settings. Many cosmetics contain known carcinogens and women working in these occupations consistently have a significantly high rate of breast cancer, based upon results of studies in mainstream medical journals and the *Journal of the National Cancer Institute.*

Beauticians have a high rate of breast cancer after only five years of on-the-job exposure to hair dyes, according to another mainstream medical journal. Considering most women are not beauticians, their exposure to these carcinogens would be less than that of the beautician; however, non-beautician women may consume enough carcinogens from hair care products over a period of longer than five years. Since effects of exposures are accumulative, this would explain the high rate of breast cancer in older women.

Beauticians have a significantly high death rate from breast cancer, revealed two studies published in mainstream medical journals. Results suggest that exposure to certain hair dyes may cause rapid spread of the more aggressive type of breast cancer. In poor African-American communities, some women perform styling and dressing of hair who are not counted in beautician statistics. A disproportionately large number of these African-American women also develop tumors that are aggressive, most often resulting in fatal breast cancer.

Women in professional, administrative, and clerical positions also have a significantly high rate of breast cancer. We believe that the frequent use of cosmetics and other personal care products are of interest for our study. We need to obtain the scientific proof to support our well-reasoned theory.

Absorption through Skin
Many women have been mistakenly led to believe that beauty aids and cosmetics do not penetrate the skin. This belief is held although it is common knowledge that drugs administered by a skin patch reach the bloodstream.

Scientific evidence proving that cosmetic ingredients enter the bloodstream through the skin follows. **Coumarin**, a carcinogen and former active ingredient in rat poison, is used in the manufacturing of **perfumes**, deodorants, shampoos, and skin fresheners often used by women and girls. Studies reveal that coumarin is readily absorbed into the bloodstream of humans upon skin contact. Coumarin, for obvious reasons, is not listed on the label of any of these products.

The National Cancer Institute showed a positive correlation between cancers and exposure to industrial plants that manufacture **perfumes**, cosmetics, and other toiletries, from an environmental study.

Alcoholic perfumes, fragrances, and colognes are often applied directly to the breast by some women. Many breast cells at the site where most malignant tumors occur receive a dosage of alcohol higher than what would be experienced by a heavy drinker. Alcohol is the main ingredient in many perfumes, fragrances, and colognes, according to the label of the manufacturers. Both scientific and medical studies confirm that alcohol is carcinogenic and that it can cause breast cancer when ingested by humans.

Some lots of alcohol used to manufacture perfumes, fragrances, colognes, and various other personal care products contain contaminants, which are linked to other cancers.

Formaldehyde and acetaldehyde are chemicals in many nail care products in widespread use by women and girls. These chemicals are known to cause cancer in experimental animals and humans. Fusel oils are present in **perfumes**, fragrances, skin creams, and body lotions. These fusel oils stimulate the body to overproduce estrogen, a promoter of cancer cells, and are implicated in **aggressive breast cancer.**

Breast Cancer Is Essentially Preventable

Consider this: in parts of Africa and rural Asia, age-adjusted incidence of breast cancer is two or three cases per 100,000 population, compared to Northern America's age-adjusted incidence of 110 cases per 100,000 population. Within five years, African and Asian women who migrated to North America or Europe—countries with a high incidence of breast cancer—their incidence of breast cancer equaled that of their new continent.

One might argue that there is something in the atmosphere of the new continent, which is causing the breast cancer. Defeating that argument is a fact that women, who are prohibited or limited to using commercial cosmetics due to religious faith and reside in the same community where incidence is high, have an age-adjusted incidence of two or three breast cancer cases per 100,000 population.

U.S. Government's Concession of Defeat Regarding a Cure

It was reported on September 18, 2000 that the National Cancer Institute conceded defeat in its efforts to find a cure for cancer, including breast cancer. Never in the history of the world has a disease been cured without finding the cause or causes; therefore, it is unlikely that within the next century, researchers will find a cure. It is of paramount importance for these studies to be carried out in order to find the major causes of breast cancer and fatal breast cancers.

Cosmetics and Breast Cancer Survivors

Carcinogens are often hidden in the list of ingredients listed as "**fragrance**." The manufacturer will most often list technical names for the carcinogenic ingredient, rendering it absolutely meaningless to many women. The International Agency for Research on Cancer publishes a list of chemicals known to cause cancers in humans. This list can be viewed at this website: http://193.51.164.11/monoeval/crthall.html.

If the average breast cancer survivor would collect her cosmetics, fragrances, and certain personal care products, placing them in a steel drum for disposal, she should hire a certified and licensed contractor to handle the toxic and hazardous waste for removal from her premises. The contractor should wear protective clothing during the removal and disposal process, due to the toxic and carcinogenic nature of many beauty aid products.

Encouraging breast cancer survivors to use cosmetics may send a message to cancer free women that beauty aid products are safe. This subliminal message is nothing more than a sophisticated marketing strategy.

Many breast cancer survivors bitterly and angrily claimed they led a healthy lifestyle, never having smoked, never drinking alcoholic beverages, exercising regularly, and eating low-fat foods high in fiber during the preliminary investigation.

These cancer victims were quite surprised when learning they'd consumed carcinogenic chemicals almost daily through their use of certain cosmetics. Many fragrances and perfumes contain an oil which causes a slow release of the scent, prolonging the life of the aroma. The downside of the use of oils is that they act in much the same way as an "estrogen patch." It also causes a consistent release of carcinogenic ingredients into the bloodstream.

Cosmetics were given to breast cancer patients, according to one woman who attended a seminar. Tobacco companies used to give away free stuff, as well.

When healthcare advocates at public forums are asked about the causes of breast cancer, the answers may include: genetic predisposition, age, high fat diet, and race. These statements are irresponsible and a disservice to the general public.

Not all girls and women who use carcinogenic products will develop breast cancer, but in view of all the foregoing scientific and medical evidence, survivors of breast cancer should proceed with great caution in using beauty aid products and cosmetics containing known carcinogens. [12]

Disclaimer: *The information contained in the Web site of the Cancer Research Center of America, Inc. (CRCA) is set forth in various mainstream medical journals that are in public domain. No representation is made, herein as to their accuracy or the method by which the results were derived. This information should in no way be construed to discredit a particular company, product or product ingredient, but should be used as a resource to enable girls and women to use the information in making informed choices as to products or ingredients they choose to use, or not use. This information may or may not be relevant to your particular concern. Cancer Research Center of America, Inc. makes no conclusions or recommendations about any company, its products and ingredients used in the manufacturing process. The information provided, herein, without a citation to a scientific or medical publication is based upon personal observations and/or personal communication. It is in no way intended to discredit or impugn the character or integrity of any organization, association, institution or individual.*

GET A WHIFF OF THIS

The following is a Press Release from the Cancer Prevention Coalition and Environmental Health Network

Press Release –
Cancer Prevention Coalition and Environmental Health Network

Perfume: Cupid's Arrow or Poison Dart?

Chicago, Feb. 8/PR Newswire – The following was released today by Samuel S. Epstein, M.D., Professor Environmental Medicine, University of Illinois School of Public Health, Chicago, and Chairman of the Cancer Prevention Coalition, and Amy Marsh, President of the Environmental Health Network, Larkspur, California:

Lovers looking for the perfect Valentine's gift should think twice before giving a bottle of toxic chemicals to their sweethearts. Recent analysis of Calvin Klein's "Eternity Eau de Parfum" (Eternity) by an industry laboratory specializing in fragrance chemistry revealed 41 ingredients. These include some known to be toxic to the skin, respiratory tract, nervous, and reproductive systems, and others known to be carcinogens; no toxicity data are available on several ingredients, while data on most are inadequate. Additionally, some ingredients are volatile and a source of indoor air pollution. Since 1995, several consumers have complained to the Food and Drug Administration (FDA) of neurological and respiratory problems due to Eternity.

The analysis was recently commissioned by the Environmental Health Network (EHN) as many members had complained of asthma, migraine, sensitization, or multiple chemical sensitivity, when exposed to Eternity.

Based on this analysis, EHN filed a Citizen Petition with the FDA on May 11, 1999, which was subsequently endorsed by the Cancer Prevention Coalition. The petition requests that the FDA take administrative action and declare Eternity "misbranded" or "adulterated" since it does not carry a warning label as required by the terms of the Food, Drug, and Cosmetic Act and the Fair Packaging and Labeling Act. Grounds for requesting the warning label include FDA regulation 21CFR Sec. 740/10: "Each ingredient used in a cosmetic product and each finished cosmetic product shall be adequately substantiated for safety prior to marketing. Any such ingredient or product whose safety is not adequately substantiated prior to marketing is misbranded unless it contains the following conspicuous statement on the principal display panel: Warning: the safety of this product has not been determined."

Since May, over 700 consumers with health problems from exposure to various mainstream fragrances have written to the FDA supporting EHN's petition. The FDA responded on November 30 to the effect that they had been unable to reach a decision on the grounds of "other priorities and the limited availability of resources." The petition is thus still open for further public complaints and endorsements.

A wide range of mainstream fragrances and perfumes, predominantly based on synthetic ingredients, are used in numerous cosmetics and toiletries, and also soaps and other household products. Currently, the fragrance industry is virtually unregulated. Its recklessness is abetted and compounded by FDA's complicity. The FDA has refused to require the industry to disclose ingredients due to trade secrecy considerations, and still takes the position that "consumers are not adversely affected—and should not be deprived of the enjoyment" of these products. The Cancer Prevention Coalition and EHN take

GET A WHIFF OF THIS

the unequivocal position that the FDA should implement its own regulations and act belatedly to protect consumer health and safety.

Valentine sweethearts should switch to organically grown (pesticide-free) roses or other flowers as safe alternatives to mainstream perfumes.[*]

Sources: Samuel S. Epstein, M.D. and Amy Marsh
Contact Feb. 8: Samuel S. Epstein, M.D., Professor of Environmental Medicine, University of Illinois, School of Public Health, Chicago, Illinois, and Chairman, the Cancer Prevention Coalition, 312-996-2297.
Contact Feb. 8: Barbara Wilkie, Environmental Health Network, P.O. Box 115, Larkspur, California 94977, 510-527-3567

---

[*] http://users.lanminds.com/~wilworks/ehnindex.html

CHAPTER 2

THE PETITION FILED AGAINST THE U.S. FDA

CONNIE PITTS

The Environmental Health Network (EHN) Petitions the Dockets Management Branch The Food and Drug Administration Department of Health and Human Services

May 7, 1999

Dockets Management Branch
The Food and Drug Administration
Department of Health and Human Services, Rm. 1–23
Rockville, MD 20857

Re: Petition to Have Fragrance Misbranded

Dear Sir or Madam:

The Environmental Health Network (EHN) petitions to have *Eternity eau de parfum* declared misbranded. EHN has selected *Eternity* for this petition because it is one of the brands we hear about the most—one that has caused drastic health problems for many, many people. *Eternity* is also representative of the type of fragrance formulation that is frequently cited as causing problems. The enclosed lab analyses, material safety data sheets, and other information clearly establish the potential dangers of many of the ingredients contained in this product. *Eternity* is manufactured by Calvin Klein Cosmetics Company, Trump Tower, 725 Fifth Avenue, New York, New York, 10022-2519, USA.

Due to the "trade-secret" status of fragrances, little information is available to the consumer as to what is in the product. The consumer is totally dependent on the integrity of the company producing the product and trusts the Food and Drug Administration (FDA) to enforce existing laws. But the ingredients in fragrances are not listed on the labels and there are no warnings. When there are no warnings on the label, the consumer naturally assumes the product has been adequately safety tested via all routes of exposure and is safe for use. Most consumers are not aware that the fragrance industry does not routinely test for neurological, respiratory, or long term effects of the materials and that most fragrance materials have only limited safety testing.

As our petition will show, this particular product contains toxic ingredients and there is no warning label. The FDA's enforcement of the required warning label on the product is essential in order for consumers to make informed choices about its safety. We feel consumers have a right to know the status of safety testing of the ingredients in products such as *Eternity* so that they might protect themselves from toxic chemicals that may cause or exacerbate acute or chronic health problems.

There are published studies that have previously identified some of the volatile organic compounds (VOCs) commonly found in fragrances and fragrance products. Widespread use of these products contributes substantially to indoor air pollution at work, home, schools, health care facilities, and recreational settings. Like tobacco smoke, the harmful chemicals currently used in these products may affect the health of many people, including:

- people with asthma and reactive airways disease who may suffer potentially fatal attacks when exposed to these products.
- people with chemical sensitivities, chronic fatigue, and other environmental illnesses.
- children, who are exposed to and harmed by the toxic chemicals found in products purchased and used by their parents, care givers and teachers.

In addition, the hazardous ingredients contained in these types of products give them the potential to be used as "inhalant" drugs by children and teenagers. This is a growing drug abuse problem and has even proved fatal. Children have already died from "huffing" air fresheners, perfumes and common household cleaners. These are products we are led to believe are safe because they are sold without warning labels.

EHN was founded over ten years ago to serve people who have been chemically injured. We receive many health complaints from people who have been exposed to chemicals used in perfumes and other fragrant consumer products. People suffer particularly in the workplace when exposed to fragrances and fragrance products because their complaints are often dismissed as frivolous (because there is a widespread misperception that fragrances are safe). Because of this, many people (including those with asthma) suffer permanent damage to their health due to fragrance products used on the job. People have become disabled by exposure to these chemicals and have lost their jobs.

In some cases, fragrance products have even been used by disgruntled co-workers and students to deliberately attack and harass those who complain about ill effects from exposure to fragrance chemicals. The case of Judith Sanderson, a high school biology teacher with reactive airway disease, is an example. She originally became ill from a formaldehyde spill in her lab, which sensitized her to other chemicals as well. Her condition deteriorated after numerous fragrance attacks from students who objected to her ban on fragrance use in her classroom. Finally, after three years, she won her right to protection and accommodation at the school through binding arbitration handled by her teacher's union (1997). At her school (in Culver City, CA), student fragrance attacks are now considered assaults.

We hope that your consideration of our petition will result in warning and ingredient labels for *Eternity* fragrance products.

Sincerely,

Amy Marsh
President

enc.

Action requested:
The petitioner requests the Commissioner to take administrative action and declare "Eternity" eau de parfum by Calvin Klein

Cosmetics Company, Trump Tower, 725 Fifth Avenue New York, NY 10022-2519 USA, misbranded.

Statement of grounds:
21CFR Sec. 740.1 states: The label of a cosmetic product shall bear a warning statement whenever necessary or appropriate to prevent a health hazard that may be associated with the product.

21CFR Sec. 740.2 states: A warning statement shall appear on the label prominently and conspicuously as compared to other words, statements, designs, or devices and in bold type on contrasting background to render it likely to be read and understood by the ordinary individual under customary conditions of purchase and use, but in no case may the letters and/or numbers be less then \1/16\ inch in height, unless an exemption pursuant to paragraph (b) of this section is established.

21CFR Sec. 740.10. Each ingredient used in a cosmetic product and each finished cosmetic product shall be adequately substantiated for safety prior to marketing. Any such ingredient or product whose safety is not adequately substantiated prior to marketing is misbranded unless it contains the following conspicuous statement of the principal display panel:

"Warning – The safety of this product has not been determined."

The perfume, "Eternity" contains substances in which the chemical, physical, and toxicological properties have not been thoroughly investigated. Many of the substances in "Eternity" have known adverse effects on health. The packaging does not carry the required warning label.

"Eternity" has been reported by consumers as having neurological and respiratory effects. (See FDA Consumer Complaints for Cosmetic Products 1995 Annual Report.) Due to the trade secret status of fragrances, fragrance ingredients are not listed on the label. This makes it extremely difficult to pinpoint substances in a fragrance that may trigger adverse reactions. Gas Chromatography studies are able to detect most of the materials in a fragrance. This testing is expensive and beyond the scope of most consumers. However, it is used routinely within the industry to develop and copy fragrance formulas. *

---

* [Excerpts from petition, under 21CFR 740.1, 740.2, 740.10 of the Federal Food, Drug, and Cosmetic Act for which authority has been delegated to the Commissioner of Food and Drugs to request the Commissioner of Food and Drugs to take administrative action. April 30, 1999, Amy Marsh, President, Environmental Health Network, P.O. Box 1155, Larkspur, CA 94977, (415) 541-5075, pg. 1–2]

Review the Chemical Analysis of Calvin Klein's Eternity Eau De Parfum

Analysis Does Not Include Ethanol, Which 25–95% May Constitute a Bottle of Perfume or Cologne.[*]

Ethanol Is a Denatured Grain Alcohol

DEFINITION of DENATURED: To make (alcohol) unfit for drinking (as by adding an obnoxious substance) without impairing usefulness for other purposes.

THE CHEMICAL ANALYSIS IS OF THE FRAGRANCE PORTION ONLY.[**]

---

[*] http://www.emedicine.com/PED/topic2715.htm
[**] The Chemical analysis was obtained from the EHN website.

GET A WHIFF OF THIS

Analysis Summary: *Eternity* eau de parfum
Huber Research (http://www.huber-research.com/)

Chemical	% of fragrance portion of formula	CAS#	Reference Material: You must register to access Aldrich MSDS information and then do a search for the chemical. Visit the web: Aldrich and Fisher are linked to those sites. EHN cannot print out that copyrighted information for you.
Ethanone, 1-(1,2,3,4,5,6,7,8-octahydro-2,3,8,8- tetramethyl-2-naphthalenyl)-	11.7	54464-57-2	A search of literature revealed very little available health or toxicology information. This compound is in common use in fragrances often at levels of 25%. (Perfumery: Practice and Principle)
Hydrocinnamaldehyde, p-tert-butyl-.alpha.-methyl-	11.6	80-54-6	Irritant. The chemical, physical, and toxicological properties have not been thoroughly investigated. This chemical is in the EPA inventory under TSCA. Label Precautions. **TARGET ORGAN DATA PATERNAL EFFECTS (TESTES, EPIDIDYMIS, SPERM DUCT)** (Aldrich)
Benzoic acid, 2-hydroxy-, phenylmethyl ester	11.1	118-58-1	Irritant. The chemical, physical, and toxicological properties have not been thoroughly investigated. (Aldrich) (Fisher)
Phthalic acid, diethyl ester	10.5	84-66-2	Irritant, CNS effects, may cause fetal effects. (Aldrich) (Fisher)
3-Buten-2-one, 4- 2,6,6-trimethyl-1-cyclohexen-1-yl)-	5.2	14901-07-6	Irritant, respiratory & skin sensitizer. The chemical, physical, and toxicological properties have not been thoroughly investigated. (Aldrich) (Fisher)
3-Cyclohexene- 1-carboxaldehyde, 4- (4-hydroxy-4-methylpntyl)-	4.8	31906-04-4	
3-Cyclohexene-1-methanol, .alph.,.alpha.,4-trimethyl-	4.2	98-55-5	Irritant. The chemical, physical, and toxicological properties have not been thoroughly investigated. (Aldrich) (Fisher)
1,3-Benzodioxole- 5-carboxaldehyde	4.0	120-57-0	Irritant, CNS effects. The chemical, physical, and toxicological properties have not been thoroughly investigated. (Aldrich) (Fisher)
Cyclopenta(g) -2-benzopyran, 1,3,4,6,7,8-hexadro- 4,6,6,7,8-hexamethyl-	3.52	1222-05-5	
Cyclopentaneacetic acid, 3-oxo-2-pentyl-, methyl ester	3.25	24851-98-7	Irritant. The chemical, physical, and toxicological properties have not been thoroughly investigated. (Aldrich)
1,6-Octadien-3-ol, 3,7-dimethyl-, acetate	3.0	115-95-7	Irritant. The chemical, physical, and toxicological properties have not been thoroughly investigated. (Aldrich)
Benzoic acid, 2-hydroxy-, (3Z)-3-hexenyl ester	3.0	65405-77-8	Irritant. The chemical, physical, and toxicological properties have not been thoroughly investigated. May be harmful by inhalation, ingestion, skin absorption. Vapor or mist is irritating to the eyes, mucous membranes and upper respiratory tract. Causes skin irritation. (Aldrich)

Compound	Value	CAS	Notes
Phenol, 2-methoxy-4-(2-propenyl) -	2.8	97-53-0	Irritant. The chemical, physical, and toxicological properties have not been thoroughly investigated. (Fisher) (Aldrich)
1,6-Nonadien-3-ol, 3,7-dimethyl-	2.4	10339-55-6	
6-Octen-1-ol, 3,7-dimethyl-	2.4	106-22-9	Severe irritant. The chemical, physical, and toxicological properties have not been thoroughly investigated. (Aldrich) (Fisher)
Oxacyclohexadecan-2-one	2.0	106-02-5	Irritant. The chemical, physical, and toxicological properties have not been thoroughly investigated. (Aldrich)
1,6-Octadien-3-ol,	3,7-dimethyl-	1.9	78-70-6	Irritant. The chemical, physical, and toxicological properties have not been thoroughly investigated. (Aldrich) (Fisher)
3-Buten-2-one, 4-(2,6,6-trimethyl-2-cyclohexen-1-yl)-	1.6	127-41-3	Irritant, skin & respiratory sensitizer. The chemical, physical, and toxicological properties have not been thoroughly investigated. (Aldrich)
Acetic acid, phenylmethyl ester	1.5	140-11-4	Toxic. May cause CNS effects, irritant, may cause cancer based upon animal studies. The chemical, physical, and toxicological properties have not been thoroughly investigated. (Aldrich) (Fisher)
2,6-Octadien-1-ol, 3,7-dimethyl-, acetate	1.0	105-87-3	The chemical, physical, and toxicological properties have not been thoroughly investigated. (Aldrich) (Fisher)
Octanol, -hydroxy-3,7-dimethyl-	.8	107-75-5	Irritant. The chemical, physical, and toxicological properties have not been thoroughly investigated. (Aldrich) (Fisher)
2-Buten-1-ol, 2-ethyl-4-(2,2,3-trimethyl- 3-cyclopenten-1-yl)-	.7	28219-61-6	The chemical, physical, and toxicological properties have not been thoroughly investigated. (Fisher)
Benzeneethanol	.49	60-12-8	Toxic, harmful by all routes, readily absorbed via skin, CNS effects. (Aldrich)
1,3-Benzodioxole, 5-(diethoxymethyl)-	.32	40527-42-2	RTECS (Registry of Toxic Effects of Chemical Substances)
1-Cyclohexene-1-butanol, 4-(diethoxymethyl)-.alpha,. alpha.-dimethyl-	.21	115217-10-2	
2-Buten-1-one, 1-(2,6,6-trimethyl-1-cyclohexen-1-yl)-	.17	23726-92-3	
Benzaldehyde, 4 -hydroxy-3-methoxy-	.15	121-33-5	Irritant. The chemical, physical, and toxicological properties have not been thoroughly investigated. (Aldrich) (Fisher)
Phenol, 2-methoxy-4-(1-propenyl)-	.15	97-54-1	Irritant. The chemical, physical, and toxicological properties have not been thoroughly investigated. (Aldrich)

GET A WHIFF OF THIS

Compound	Amount	CAS	Notes
Oxacycloheptadec-10-en-2-one	.13	28645-51-4	
2-Octanol, 8,8-diethoxy-2,6-dimethyl-	.12	7779-94-4	
2-Propen-1-ol, 3-phenyl-	.08	104-54-1	Irritant. The chemical, physical, and toxicological properties have not been thoroughly investigated. (Aldrich) (Fisher)
6-Octen-3-ol, 3,7-dimethyl-, acetate	.08	50373-60-9	
6-Octen-3-ol, 3,7-dimethyl-	.07	18479-51-1	
7-Octen-4-one, 2,6-dimethyl-	.07	1879-00-1	
Acetic acid, (cyclohexyloxy)-, 2-propenyl ester	.06	68901-15-5	
2,6-Octadien-1-ol, 3,7-dimethyl-	.05	106-25-2	Irritant. The chemical, physical, and toxicological properties have not been thoroughly investigated. (Aldrich)
Phenol, 2,6-bis(1,1-dimethylethyl)-4-methyl-	.05	128-37-0	Irritant, cancer suspect agent, may cause reproductive/fetal effects. The chemical, physical, and toxicological properties have not been thoroughly investigated. (Aldrich) (Fisher)
Benzaldehyde, 4-methoxy-	.04	123-11-5	Irritant. The chemical, physical, and toxicological properties have not been thoroughly investigated. (Aldrich) (Fisher)
Benzenemethanol	.04	100-51-6	Irritant, skin sensitizer, CNS effect, harmful by all routes of exposure. (Aldrich) (Fisher)
1,3,6-Octatriene, 3,7-dimethyl-	.04	29714-87-2	The chemical, physical, and toxicological properties have not been thoroughly investigated. (Aldrich)
Benzoic acid, 2-hydroxy-, ethyl ester	.02	118-61-6	Irritant. The chemical, physical, and toxicological properties have not been thoroughly investigated. (Aldrich) (Fisher)

Responses to the Petition

Despite lack of media attention, there have been over 1,300 responses.

You will notice there are no written signatures on letters sent to the FDA via e-mail.

All the letters I'm sharing were obtained from EHN's website.

To view additional responses, please read:

http://users.lmi.net/~wilworks/FDApetition/bkgrinfo.htm

November 6, 1999

Dockets Management Branch
The Food and Drug Administration
Department of Health and Human Services, Rm. 1–23
12420 Parklawn Dr.
Rockville, MD 20857

via fax: 301.827.6870

RE: Docket Number: **99P-1340/CP 1**
Petition FDA to declare Calvin Klein's *Eternity eau de parfum* "misbranded"

To Whom It May Concern:

Perfumes contain hundreds of lipophilic solvents. When a lipophilic solvent is applied to the surface of the skin (or inhaled) it is absorbed into the bloodstream and carried into the brain, liver and kidneys, and stored in fatty tissues throughout the body. **As far as perfumes are concerned, what goes on the skin goes through the skin. This is the reality of the situation.**

It is only logical that perfumes and their transdermal "delivery system" should be subjected to the same rigorous testing and safety requirements that the FDA already applies to skin-patch drug delivery systems. Most of the drugs that the FDA tests for patch-delivery have already been approved for delivery into the body by other means, whereas perfume components have neither been investigated nor approved for delivery by *any* means. We don't even know their effects, much less what concentrations are building up in the body.

Also to be taken into account is the fact that the human respiratory system is an extremely efficient absorber of volatile organic compounds. Approximately 95 percent of the volatile organics that are inhaled are absorbed into the body.

The use of perfume constitutes the delivery of harmful phthalates, phenols and potential hormone disrupters as well as dozens of sensitizing and/or hazardous organic solvents—all with unknown long-term effects—into persistent storage within organs and fat depots of the body. Undoubtedly some degree of neurotoxicity or poisoning is caused by perfume ingredients. Therefore perfumes (especially the modern designer perfumes) should be considered dangerous until proven safe.

It is time to go beyond ignorance and wishful thinking. The first step is to conduct tests to investigate the appearance of perfume components in blood and fatty tissue after skin and lung exposure. It is outrageous to not be carefully testing the effects of repeatedly dosing the body with a solution containing hundreds of organic solvents of unknown long-term effects—particularly in these times of increasing cancer rates. Grandfathering is no excuse for not doing these tests. Neither is the "self-regulation" of the perfume industry. Safety testing by vested interests is meaningless.

The fragrance industry has argued for years that levels are so low they don't matter. Well, let us do the experiments and see what the levels are and what damage those levels produce. Determine the reality of: 1) the residual concentration of perfume components; 2) the build-up of this concentration with repeated use; and 3) the long-term effects of these concentrations, with particular attention to increased risk of breast cancer in women who are regular users of perfumes.

Sincerely,

Richard H. Conrad, PhD Biochemist

GET A WHIFF OF THIS

50

Anderson Laboratories, Inc.
P. O. Box 323
773 Main Street
West Hartford, VT 05084
Tel 802-295-7344
www.andersonlaboratories.com

1120 '99 JUN -8 A9:33

June 3, 1999

Dockets Management Branch
FDA
Dept HHS
Rm 1-23
12420 Parklawn Dr.
Rockville MD 20857

Regarding Docket 99P-1340/CP 1 Petition concerning Clavin Klein's Eternity

We support the petition regarding a need for a hazard warning on "eau de parfum."

Our independent laboratory research demonstrated that several typical eau de parfum's have readily demonstrated toxic properties. When mice breathed these vapors, they developed a number of signs of neurotoxicity (tremors, loss of balance, twitching, abnormal repetitive movements, altered posture and gait, etc.); some were so severely damaged they died as a result of breathing these fragrance products. Mice also developed decreased expiratory airflow as if they were having an asthmatic attack while breathing the eau de parfum (these were normal mice just prior to their exposures to these fragrance products).

These findings are summarized in the enclosed scientific article "Acute toxic effects of fragrance products" (which was published in a peer-reviewed scientific journal). We also have documented these neurotoxic effects on a video tape which we could make available to you if you desire.

Julius Anderson, M.D. Ph.D.
Vice President, Anderson Laboratories.

99P-1340

C93

CONNIE PITTS

Dockets Management Branch
The Food and Drug Administration
Department of Health and Human Services, Rm. 1–23
12420 Parklawn Dr.
Rockville, MD 20857

FAX: 310-827-6870
E-mail: mailto:fdadockets@oc.fda.gov

Re: Petition filed with the FDA to have "Eternity" by Calvin Klein declared misbranded.
Docket Number: **99P-1340/CP 1**

This is a comment on the specific case of the "Eternity" perfume, but this case has more general implications for the following reasons:

1. Perfumes and perfumed products are a well-demonstrated cause of asthma.
2. The incidence of asthma and deaths from asthma have been rising dramatically in recent decades.
3. The use of perfumed consumer products has been rising dramatically in recent decades.
4. A reasonable supposition can be made that perfume and perfumed products account for some of this rise in morbidity and mortality, possibly accounting for a major part of the rise.

The issue is a complex one, from scientific, regulatory and intellectual property perspectives. I bring some important perspectives to this matter as a physician/scientist on the faculty of Harvard Medical School, an individual with mild—moderate asthma, one who has written publicly on chemical safety regulatory matters (e.g. *Wall Street Journal* 9 July 91) and one who holds copyrights and has patents submitted.

The scientific complexity arises here from the multiplicity of ingredients in perfumes, often several hundred. It is likely that the large majority of ingredients in any one perfume are not significant triggers of asthma. However, from my own personal and clinical experience and from review of the literature, it appears that many, but not all perfumes and perfumed consumer products do trigger asthma. Judging from this information, it appears likely that only a small number of ingredients in perfumes are significant triggers of asthma. However, these ingredients are not well characterized and are certainly unknown to members of the general population. Unfortunately, the correlation between odorous ingredients of a perfume and asthma-triggering ingredients is poor, and the time before onset of symptoms can be minutes to hours the consumer and others exposed to the consumer's products do not have much basis for identifying or avoiding the hazards themselves.

For the asthma sufferer, this matter is as serious as exposure to other asthma triggers such as smoke. Yet, because the perfume constituents responsible for asthma are so poorly identified or disclosed, the asthma-sufferer does not have the same ability to avoid the asthma trigger. The matter is a complex one because the responsibilities for this type of pollution overlap between the FDA, EPA and OSHA and other agencies. The jurisdictional complexity arises from the multiplicity of situations in which perfumed products are used:

1. By individuals with asthma
2. By second-hand exposure from parents and day-care workers
3. As occupational issues from use in workplaces and hotels.

Yet, we cannot allow this regulatory complexity to deter us from acting in face of the rising epidemic of asthma that we face.

I propose the following as a minimum for this product and for others:

A. The product should bear a hazard label warning that the ingredients have not been tested and are suspected of causing asthma.
B. To bear a different label, a product could go through a certification process in which propensity to trigger asthma would be judged.

A more satisfactory general solution would be:

C. To catalog and severely restrict the perfume ingredients which trigger asthma.

There are difficulties in that the nature of many ingredients is protected as trade secrets, but this should not prevent the use of mass spectroscopy and related techniques to catalog relevant ingredients that are common or most linked to asthma.

The incidence of asthma is increasing, and the problem preferentially afflicts some groups such as inner city residents, who appear to use perfumed products out of proportion to the use in the general population. Action must be taken. I have spoken out publicly on issues in which too much regulation has been applied to health problems; the issue here is the opposite: there is a failure to act when action is needed. It would be tragic if protection from volatile asthma-triggering chemicals were to fall between the cracks of jurisdiction of different agencies.

Michael M. Segal MD, PhD
Assistant Professor of Surgery
Harvard Medical School

GET A WHIFF OF THIS

Wednesday, September 29, 1999

Dockets Management Branch
The Food and Drug Administration
Department of Health and Human Services, Rm. 1–23
12420 Parklawn Dr.
Rockville, MD 20857

by email: mailto:fdadockets@oc.fda.gov

Dear Food and Drug Administration:

I'm writing to petition your Administration to declare *Eternity* eau de parfum "misbranded," as a comment to Docket Number "99P-1340/CP 1." The basis of this petition is the lack of a warning label on the product informing consumers that all the materials in the product, and the product itself, have not been adequately tested for safety. Independent laboratory analysis of this product has revealed such chemicals as diethyl phthalate (suspected hormone disrupter with ability to accumulate in the fatty tissues of the human body through skin absorption); phenols (suspected carcinogens, may cause reproductive harm); benzoethanol (rated toxic, readily absorbed via skin, central nervous system effects); musks xylene and musk ketone (recently in the news as suspected carcinogens which accumulate in human and animal tissues) and skin and respiratory irritants.

As a citizen, I have (or ought to have) a civil right to breathe clean air. I also should have the right to know what's in that air whenever feasible. When someone douses themselves with artificial cologne or perfume, I am denied those rights. I also believe that all ingredients should be listed on any food, drug, or any product ingested, absorbed, or applied to the body. Consumers ought to have an informed choice about what goes in or on their bodies. Unfortunately, the law states that only certain chemicals have to be listed on the label, and that "fragrances" are protected from disclosure by Confidential Business Information, (CBI). However, CBI does not shield disclosure of substances that are known hazards (or should be known). Inadequate safety testing is no excuse for not labeling a hazardous ingredient or misbranding a product.

I urge your administration to do a more thorough analysis of Calvin Klein's "Eternity Eau de Parfum." Should your analysis confirm any of the results of independent studies it seems appropriate that this product ought not be allowed onto the market. Perfume manufactures could and should reformulate, because public health always comes first.

Sincerely,

Blake Brown
Sierra Club, San Francisco Bay Chapter
Toxics Committee Chair

Sat, 14 Aug 1999

Dockets Management Branch
The Food and Drug Administration
Department of Health and Human Services, Rm. 1–23
12420 Parklawn Dr.
Rockville, MD 20857

Re: 99P-1340/CP 1
Petition to Have *Eternity eau de parfum* Misbranded

Dear Sir or Madam:

In May, 1999, the Environmental Health Network (EHN) submitted the above petition to have Calvin Klein's *Eternity eau de parfum* declared misbranded. I am writing because I fully support this petition and request that the FDA give it careful attention with regard to your regulations 21CFR Sec. 740.1, 21CFR Sec. 740.2, and 21CFR Sec. 740.10. Regulation 21CFR Sec. 740.10 specifically states:

> Each ingredient used in a cosmetic product and each finished cosmetic product shall be adequately substantiated for safety prior to marketing. Any such ingredient or product whose safety is not adequately substantiated prior to marketing is misbranded unless it contains the following conspicuous statement on the principal display panel:
>
> "Warning – The safety of this product has not been determined."

As the petition shows, *Eternity* contains toxic ingredients and ingredients whose safety have not been substantiated. There is no warning label on its packaging.

We all have a right to know the status of safety testing of the ingredients in products such as *Eternity* so that we can protect ourselves and our families from toxic chemicals that may cause health problems. Most people are not aware that most fragrance materials have only limited safety testing. They wrongfully assume these products are safe to use in any setting and are surprised when people complain.

Like tobacco smoke, the harmful chemicals currently used in these products may effect the health of many people, including people with asthma, chemical sensitivities, chronic fatigue, and other environmental illnesses. Children are particularly vulnerable to toxic chemicals found in products purchased and used by their parents, care givers and teachers.

Please act on behalf of the millions of people who have suffered physical illness and injury resulting from fragrance exposure at work, at school and in social settings. These toxic chemicals act as powerful barriers to people disabled by asthma and chemical sensitivities. Because of this, toxic chemicals in fragrances have already ruined countless lives. Thank you.

Sincerely yours,

Lawrence A. Plumlee, M.D., President CSDA
(Chemical Sensitivity Disorders Association)

June 11, 1999

Dockets Management Branch
Food and Drug Administration
Department of Health and Human Services, Room 1–23
12420 Parklawn Drive
Rockville, MD 20852-1745

Re: DOCKET #99P-1340/CP 1

Dear Sir or Madam:

I am writing about a public health matter that effects not only the thousands of people who are chemically sensitive but those with asthma and chronic fatigue; the elderly and the very young; those undergoing chemotherapy; and many Gulf War veterans. We are all affected by synthetic chemicals in fragrance products. "Dear Abby" has published several letters (probably representative of many more) from people who experienced headaches or respiratory difficulties from inadvertent exposures to fragranced products. In 1989 a New York woman sprayed with a perfume by a Bloomingdale's salesperson won her lawsuit against the store, after she spent eleven days in a hospital in critical condition.

The above petition asks for a much-needed warning to potential users of at least one fragrance. Though most of us know that cosmetics are the least regulated of those substances under the jurisdiction of the FDA, several of your regulations do apply: 21CFR Sec. 740.1, 21CFR Sec. 740.2, and 21CFR Sec. 740.10. The latter states:

> Each ingredient used in a cosmetic product and each finished cosmetic product shall be adequately substantiated for safety prior to marketing. Any such ingredient or product whose safety is not adequately substantiated prior to marketing is misbranded unless it contains the following conspicuous statement on the principal display panel:

"Warning—The safety of this product has not been determined."

The petition shows that Eternity contains toxic ingredients and ingredients whose safety have not been substantiated, yet there is no warning label on its packaging. How are we to know which fragranced products may have adverse effects on our health if there are no warning labels?

Besides Eternity, I have pinpointed several other perfumes as giving me trouble. There are plenty of others that I've not been able to identify. I shudder to think what encounters with any of these perfumes are doing to babies.

Please help prevent such reactions in the millions of people who are exposed to these untested, unlabeled substances every day, at home, at work, at school, and at social gatherings. Thank you.

Sincerely,

Lynn Lawson, Chair, Public Relations

cc: Senator Richard Durbin
    Senator Peter Fitzgerald
    Representative Jan Schakowsky
    Chicago Tribune
    Chicago Sun-Times
    Ralph Nader (Public Citizen)
    [U.S.] Access Board
    Illinois Public Health Advocate
    Greenpeace
    Center for Health, Environment, and Justice
    The Alliance for Democracy
    American Lung Association
    Environmental Health Network [shared w/FPIN w/permission]

GET A WHIFF OF THIS

June 8, 1999

Dockets Management Branch
The Food and Drug Administration
Department of Health and Human Services, Rm. 1–23
12420 Parklawn Dr.
Rockville, MD 20857

Re: 99P-1340/CP 1
Petition to Have *Eternity* eau de pafum declared "Misbranded."

Dear Sir or Madam:

As president of the Environmental Health Network, the sponsoring organization for the above petition, I have already sent you a letter on behalf of our board of directors. I wish to add my own comments here as a private citizen. I urge your thoughtful and lawful consideration of the contents of this petition, as mandated by your own regulations 21CFR Sec. 740.1, 21CFR Sec. 740.2, and 21CFR Sec. 740.10.

Perhaps you will understand the urgency of our petition in this context. Several decades ago, people protesting against public tobacco use were ignored and ridiculed, treated as crackpots or lunatics. They were in a position similar to those people today who are suffering from the effects of widespread, public fragrance use and who are trying desperately to be heard by anyone who could be of help. Complaints sent to doctors, medical associations, employers, government agencies, newspaper editors, even to the fragrance industry itself, are almost universally ignored.

Like tobacco smoke, fragrances and fragrance products containing synthetic chemicals:

- are marketed to people who want to feel glamorous, sexy and "cool;"

- are often repeatedly used throughout the day, allowing small amounts of harmful substances to be absorbed into the users' body;
- cause harm to other people in the immediate vicinity, through "off-gassing" of toxic fumes. These fumes are immediately harmful to people with asthma and multiple chemical sensitivities (MCS); and
- cause immediate deterioration of air quality, indoors and out.

In addition to being health hazards, tobacco smoke and heavy fragrances are often considered unpleasant and annoying in public settings—not glamorous or cool at all. People who do not use these products themselves often object to being forced into smelling them at restaurants, theaters, other recreational settings, and in the workplace and at schools.

You don't have to have asthma or MCS to object to tasting *Eternity* instead of your sushi, or to smelling *Giorgio* instead of wholesome fresh air.

Unfortunately, people who use these products often insist they have a "right" to use them in any setting, regardless of how unpleasant or dangerous these products may be for themselves or anyone else. Ironically, thanks to a massive public education campaign and regulations against smoking in many public settings, many smokers have become far more considerate than most fragrance users.

There are other parallels I must mention. Like the tobacco industry, the fragrance industry has attempted to gain a foothold with teens and children. Miss Piggy, of Muppet fame, has her own signature fragrance, *Moi*.

You can't tell me this is a product designed to appeal to a supposedly sophisticated adult. No, Miss Piggy has become the Joe Camel of the fragrance industry—and Jim Hensen, her creator, if still alive, would be writhing with shame if he knew what harmful substances are polluting the lungs and fatty tissues of her innocent fans as a result.

Parents who are otherwise extremely cautious about food, clothing and other products they purchase for their children enthusiastically buy synthetically scented lotions, shampoos, baby wipes, diapers and even toys. (I saw a vanilla scented ball for toddlers in a Discovery Toys catalog just yesterday.) Even children with asthma are subjected to these products. This is because the parents are lulled into thinking these products are safe. They are readily available and there are no warning labels.

This is a tragedy in the making, and even more tragic for being preventable. I live in a neighborhood with many new families. I see so many small children at the mercy of an adult reeking of neurotoxic fragrance chemicals. When do these children ever get to breathe real fresh air? Their parents and babysitters are scented and toxic, their homes are full of "air fresheners" and scented cosmetics and cleaning products. Even their clothing is contaminated by heavily scented dryer sheets and detergents. I fear for the health of these children, who are absorbing these chemicals through their lungs and skin. I fear that asthma, brain damage, chemical sensitivies, allergies, and behavioral and learning difficulties will be the inevitable result. Perhaps even the increase in childhood cancers might be partially related to this unrelenting exposure to toxic chemicals and chemical combinations.

I am aware of several studies on the toxicity of fragrance products, but to my knowledge they have not been published in pediatric journals. Even though the American Medical Association and the American Lung Association now list fragrances as "asthma triggers," I wonder how many doctors have time to search these websites. Certainly the HMO I belong to is not notifying new parents or asthma patients about the hazards of these products.

In conclusion, tobacco and fragrance products are both manufactured by industries who would prefer not to be held accountable for the adverse effects of their products. These industries spend considerable amounts of time and energy influencing the general public and public servants through advertising, lobbying, and questionable "scientific studies" paid for by industry groups. Like the tobacco industry in the not so distant past, I suspect the fragrance industry has been suppressing information and is now playing for time—hoping to rake in as much profit as possible before facing the inevitable results of its careless and deliberate erosion of public health.

Please act to restore and protect the health of the American public, and make this petition a priority. My own experience, and that of many other people I have spoken with, tells me that most fragrance products are currently dangerous. Consumers need to be warned, and the industry needs to develop safe formulations.

Sincerely,

Amy Marsh

GET A WHIFF OF THIS

Responding to the Petition

You may respond to the petition by writing to:

Dockets Management Branch
The Food and Drug Administration
Department of Health and Human Services, Rm. 1–23
12420 Parklawn Dr.
Rockville, MD 20857

Or via email: mailto:fdadockets@oc.fda.gov

Mention Docket # 99P-1340/CP-1
(If using email, please place docket number in subject line.)

Example of what to say:

I fully support the petition to have Calvin Klein's "Eternity eau de parfum" declared misbranded.

Please include your name, address, and telephone number. It's that simple.

CHAPTER 3

PERFUMES POSE SERIOUS HEALTH RISKS

CONNIE PITTS

JULIA KENDALL GRANTED PERMISSION FOR HER WORK TO BE COPIED AND SHARED FOR THE PURPOSE OF EDUCATING OTHERS.

Anyone may copy or share Julia's work—just be sure to credit Julia Kendall.

Thank you, Julia.
Your work lives on.

Health Risks from Perfumes:
The Twenty Most Common Chemicals Found In Thirty-One Fragrance Products by a 1991 EPA Study

By Julia Kendall (1995)[*]

Compiled by Julia Kendall, Co-Chair, Citizens for a Toxic-Free Marin. Reference: Lance Wallace, Environmental Protection Agency; Phone (703) 341-7509

Symptoms of exposure are taken from industry-generated Material Safety Data Sheets (MSDS).

Principal chemicals found in scented products are:

ACETONE
(In: cologne, dishwashing liquid and detergent, nail enamel remover) – On **EPA, RCRA, CERCLA Hazardous Waste lists.** "inhalation can cause dryness of the mouth and throat, dizziness, nausea, incoordination, slurred speech, drowsiness, and, in severe exposures, coma." "Acts primarily as a central nervous system (CNS) depressant."

BENZALDEHYDE
(In: perfume, cologne, hairspray, laundry bleach, deodorants, detergent, vaseline lotion, shaving cream, shampoo, bar soap, dishwasher detergent) – Narcotic. Sensitizer. "Local anesthetic, CNS depressant . . . irritation to the mouth, throat, eyes, skin, lungs, and GI tract causing nausea and abdominal pain." "May cause kidney damage." "Do not use with contact lenses."

BENZYL ACETATE
(In: perfume, cologne, shampoo, fabric softener, stickup air freshener, dishwashing liquid and detergent, soap, hairspray, bleach, after shave,

---

[*] Julia Kendall died July 12, 1997 from Multiple Chemical Sensitivities and Leukemia caused by Malathion (pesticide) poisoning.

GET A WHIFF OF THIS

deodorants) – Carcinogenic (linked to pancreatic cancer); "From vapors: irritating to eyes and respiratory passages, exciting cough." "In mice: hyperaemia of the lungs." Can be absorbed through the skin, causing systemic effects. "Do not flush to sewer."

BENZYL ALCOHOL
(In: perfume, cologne, soap, shampoo, nail enamel remover, air freshener, laundry bleach and detergent, vaseline lotion, deodorants, fabric softener) – "irritating to the upper respiratory tract" . . . "headache, nausea, vomiting, dizziness, drop in blood pressure, CNS depression, and death in severe cases due to respiratory failure."

CAMPHOR
(In: perfume, shaving cream, nail enamel, fabric softener, dishwasher detergent, nail color, stickup air freshener) – "local irritant and CNS stimulant" . . . "readily absorbed through body tissues" . . . "irritation of eyes, nose and throat" . . . "dizziness, confusion, nausea, twitching muscles and convulsions" "Avoid inhalation of vapors."

ETHANOL
(In: perfume, hairspray, shampoo, fabric softener, dishwashing liquid and detergent, laundry detergent, shaving cream, soap, vaseline lotion, air fresheners, nail color and remover, paint and varnish remover) – **On EPA Hazardous Waste list.** Symptoms: ". . . fatigue, irritating to eyes and upper respiratory tract even in low concentrations . . ." "inhalation of ethanol vapors can have effects similar to those characteristic of ingestion. These include an initial stimulatory effect, followed by drowsiness, impaired vision, ataxia, stupor." Causes CNS disorder.

ETHYL ACETATE
(In: after shave, cologne, perfume, shampoo, nail enamel remover, fabric softener, dishwashing liquid) – Narcotic. **On EPA Hazardous Waste list.** ". . . irritating to the eyes and respiratory tract" . . . "may cause headache and narcosis [stupor]" . . . "defatting effect on skin and may cause drying and cracking" . . . "may cause anemia with leukocytosis and damage to liver and kidneys" "Wash thoroughly after handling."

LIMONENE
(In: perfume, cologne, disinfectant spray, bar soap, shaving cream, deodorants, nail color and remover, fabric softener, dishwashing liquid, air fresheners, after shave, bleach, paint and varnish remover) – Carcinogenic. "Prevent its contact with skin or eyes because it is an irritant and sensitizer." "Always wash thoroughly after using this material and before eating, drinking . . . applying cosmetics. Do not inhale limonene vapor."

LINALOOL
(In: perfume, cologne, bar soap, shampoo, hand lotion, nail enamel remover, hairspray, laundry detergent, dishwashing liquid, vaseline lotion, air fresheners, bleach powder, fabric softener, shaving cream, after shave, solid deodorant) – Narcotic . . . "respiratory disturbances" . . . "Attracts bees." "In animal tests: ataxic gait, reduced spontaneous motor activity and depression . . . development of respiratory disturbances leading to death" . . . "depressed frog-heart activity." Causes CNS disorder.

METHYLENE CHLORIDE
(In: shampoo, cologne, paint and varnish remover) – **Banned by the FDA in 1988!** No enforcement possible due to trade secret laws protecting chemical fragrance industry. **On EPA, RCRA, CERCLA Hazardous Waste lists.** "Carcinogenic" . . . "Absorbed, stored in body fat, it metabolizes to carbon monoxide, reducing oxygen-carrying capacity of the blood." "Headache, giddiness, stupor, irritability, fatigue, tingling in the limbs." Causes CNS disorders.

a-PINENE
(In: bar and liquid soap, cologne, perfume, shaving cream, deodorants, dishwashing liquid, air freshener) – Sensitizer [damaging to the immune system].

g-TERPINENE
(In: cologne, perfume, soap, shaving cream, deodorant, air freshener) – "Causes asthma and CNS disorders."

GET A WHIFF OF THIS

a-TERPINEOL
(In: perfume, cologne, laundry detergent, bleach powder, laundry bleach, fabric softener, stick-up air freshener, vaseline lotion, cologne, soap, hairspray, after shave, roll-on deodorant) – "highly irritating to mucous membranes" . . . "Aspiration into the lungs can produce pneumonitis of even fatal edema." Can also cause "excitement, ataxia [loss of muscular coordination], hypothermia, CNS and respiratory depression, and headache." "Prevent repeated or prolonged skin contact."

Unable to secure MSDS for the following chemicals: 1,8-CINEOLE; B-CITRONELLOL; b-MYRCENE; NEROL; OCIMENE; b-PHENETHYL ALCOHOL; a-TERPINOLENE.*

FABRIC SOFTENERS – HEALTH RISKS
From Dryer Exhaust and Treated Fabrics

Chemicals found in fabric softeners by U.S. Environmental Protection Agency (EPA)

In addition to Alpha-Terpineol, Benzyl Acetate, Benzyl Alcohol, Camphor, Ethyl Acetate, Limonene and Linalool, all mentioned above in the Twenty Most Common Chemicals Found in Thirty-One Fragrance Products, **fabric softeners** also contain:

CHLOROFORM – Neurotoxic. Anesthetic. Carcinogen. On **EPA's Hazardous Waste list.** "Avoid contact with eyes, skin, clothing. Do not breathe vapors . . . Inhalation of vapors may cause headache, nausea, vomiting, dizziness, drowsiness, irritation of respiratory tract and loss of consciousness." "Inhalation can be fatal." "Chronic effects of overexposure may include kidney and/or liver damage." "Medical conditions generally aggravated by exposure: kidney disorders, liver disorders, heart disorders, skin disorders." "Conditions to avoid: **HEAT** . . ." Listed on California's Proposition 65.

---

* References: Material Safety Data Sheets [MSDS]. Distributed by the Environmental Health Network (of California), with permission of Julia Kendall. (http://users.lmi.net/~wilworks/ehn20.htm)
Note: Flyers can be printed from EHN's website.

PENTANE – "Danger—Harmful if inhaled; extremely flammable. Keep away from heat . . . Avoid breathing vapor." "Inhalation of vapors may cause headache, nausea, vomiting, dizziness, drowsiness, irritation of respiratory tract and loss of consciousness. Repeated inhalation of vapors may cause central nervous system depression. Contact can cause eye irritation. Prolonged exposure may cause dermatitis (skin rash)."

Fabric softeners, like other fragrant products, contain petrochemicals, used in untested combinations. These chemicals can adversely affect the central nervous system (CNS)—your brain and spine.

CNS exposure symptoms include: aphasia, blurred vision, disorientation, dizziness, headaches, hunger, memory loss, numbness in face, and pain in neck and spine. CNS disorders include: Alzheimer's Disease, Attention Deficit Disorder, Dementia, Multiple Chemical Sensitivity, Multiple Sclerosis, Parkinson's Disease, Seizures, Strokes, and Sudden Infant Death Syndrome (SIDS)

If you use fabric softeners (liquid or sheets), **STOP.**

- Save the container as evidence—doctors can request analysis.
- If made ill by fabric softener used by another person, give product name if known.
- Provide a description of your symptoms
- Take this information to your doctor to help document your symptoms.[*]

ACT NOW

If you suffer symptoms from exposures to fabric softeners:

* Telephone 1-800-638-2772, press 1, then press 999 to file an official complaint with the U.S. Consumer Product Safety

---

[*] (Flyers can be printed online: http://users.lanminds.com/~wilworks/ehnfs.htm)

Commission. Say you want to file a report on a hazardous product. **Emphasize central nervous system disorder symptoms.**

Allergic symptoms are not given priority in Commission investigations. Demand a recall. Please have everyone you know who reacts to fabric softeners call. The tally will be useful in litigation and publicity.

* Telephone 1-301-504-0424—consumer product reports are available (for a fee) under the Freedom of Information Act. Request any of the following:

    1. Emergency Room reports
    2. Death Certificate reports
    3. Consumer Complaints
    4. In-depth Investigations

* Telephone 1-800-543-1745 – Proctor and Gamble *(Downy & Bounce)*; 1-800-598-5005 – Lever Bros. *(Snuggle)*; or, contact the manufacturer of the product that you know makes you ill.

* Call the Air Quality Management and the Air Resources agencies in your area. File a complaint. Request a list of their board members. Ask for information regarding their policies for presenting issues to their boards. Request the boards consider the issue of scented fabric softeners in dryer exhausts as a factor in outdoor air pollution—fragrance products are made with petrochemicals used in untested combinations.[*]

---

[*] http://users.lmi.net/~wilworks/ehnfs.htm
Note: Flyers can be printed from EHN's website.

Making Sense of Scents
Compiled by Julia Kendall

A few chemicals in fragrances known to be neurotoxic, hexachlorophene; acetyl-ethyl-tetramethyl-tetralin; zinc-pyridinethione; 2,4,dinitro-3-methyl-6-tert-butylanisole; 1-Butanol; 2-butanol; tert-Butanol; Isobutanol; t-Butyl Toluene. Neurotoxic properties of chemicals found in fragrances have caused testicular atrophy in lab animals as well as myelin disease. The myelin sheath protects the nerves and does not regenerate. (Compiled from TOXLINE databases of fragrances industry and medical journals.)

Multiple Sclerosis, Parkinson's, Lupus and Alzheimer's are all neurological disorders. Dyslexia is a neurological dysfunction. Could any of these neurological dysfunctions be caused by exposure to neurotoxic chemicals? Symptoms are often identical to chemical hypersensitivity. Sudden Infant Death Syndrome (SIDS) is also a neurological dysfunction. **Could fragrant fabric softeners or detergents emitting neurotoxic chemicals cause the neurological breakdown?**

Limonene, also listed as one of the 20 most common chemicals in fragrances, is a known carcinogen. The Merck Index cautions that Limonene is a sensitizer. Sensitizers have the capacity to cause Multiple Chemical Sensitivities (MCS).

Benzaldehyde, also one of the most common chemicals in the EPA's fragrance study, is a sensitizer. It is also a narcotic, according to the Merck Index.

A few chemicals found in fragrances known to cause cancer and birth defects: methylene chloride; toluene; methyl ethyl ketone; methyl isobutyl ketone, tert Butyl; sec Butyl; benzyl chloride. (Compiled by comparing a list of 120 fragrance chemicals from the EPA, obtained through the Freedom of Information Act and California's Prop 65 List of Chemicals.)

A few chemicals found in fragrances designated as hazardous waste disposal chemicals: methylene chloride, toluene, meythl ethyl

GET A WHIFF OF THIS

ketone, ethanol, benzal chloride. These chemicals are listed in the EPA's Code 40 of Federal Regulations, Ch 1, Section 261.33.

In a National Institute of Occupational Safety and Health study conducted by Syracuse Research Corporation, Report No. SRC TR 81-521,1981, benzoin is named as a chemical used in fragrances found to cause enlarged lymph nodes in both male and female mice and enlarged spleens in males. Liver damage is also cited.

National Institutes of Health, "Issues and Challenges in Environmental Health," NIH Pub #87-861 . . . "Allergic reactions and hypersensitivity diseases, for instance, are among the most costly of U.S. health problems afflicting at least 35,000,000 Americans."

Article "One Woman's Perfume—Another Woman's Poison" in *Let's Live,* "The chief reactions we see are those that affect the nervous system—headaches, anxiety, and depression. There are two major ways in which cosmetics and their chemical constituents can affect the body. One is through direct contact. Inhalation is the other major route for molecules of an active substance to enter the blood stream. "There is a route from the nasal passage into the nervous system," says Mandall. "It is the way, for instance, that inhaled cocaine has an effect on the brain."

THE LAW
The Americans with Disabilities Act of 1992 guarantees access for the disabled to institutions, such as government agencies, libraries, doctors' offices, retail stores, and many others. Multiple Chemical Sensitivity/Environmental Illness is recognized as a disability by The Social Security Administration and HUD. Fragrances are a "barrier to access" to MCS/EI disabled, since breathing is affected. Breathing is a "major life activity" as defined by the ADA. Fragrance bans meet the "reasonable accommodation" clause of the ADA, since elimination and substitution are not expensive.

Postal Regulations, Domestic Mail Manual, 124.395 Fragrance Advertising Samples (39 USC 3001 (g) April 1990) states that fragrance strips for mailing "cannot be activated except by opening a glued flap or binder or by removing an overlying ply of paper."

California AB 2709 (as of January 1, 1992) states that "fragrances contained in any newspaper, magazine, or other periodically-printed material, published or offered for sale, or contained in any advertisement—mailed or otherwise distributed—shall be enclosed in a sealant sufficient to protect a consumer from inadvertent exposure to the cosmetic—including, but not limited to, the inadvertent inhalation thereof."

[Excerpts from Making Sense of Scents]

Compiled by the late Julia Kendall, Co-Chair for a Toxic-Free Marin, borrowing from Irene Wilkenfeld's "Fragrance Facts," and from research contributed by Karen Stevens, Carol Kuczora, Milan Param, Richard Conrad PhD, Susan Nordmark, Susan Springer, Mary Ann Handrus, Susan Molloy, and Sandy Ross PhD., distributed by EHN.[*]

---

[*] http://users.lmi.net/~wilworks/ehnmsofs.htm
Note: Barb Wilke, President of EHN, has updated some information on this site. Feel free to copy and post, crediting Julia Kendall.

Fragrance Chemicals as Toxic Substances

Citizens for a Safe Learning Environment
Halifax, Nova Scotia

The chemicals Acetone, Benzaldehyde, Benzyl Acetate, Benzyl Alcohol, Camphor, Ethanol, Limomene, Linalool, Methylene chloride (dichloromethane) and a-Terpineol are listed in the full text of this article. Since I have already included information regarding these chemicals in Twenty Most Common Chemicals Found in Thirty-one Fragrance Products and Fabric Softeners—Health Risks, I would like to share the following, summarized from the writing of Sandra Moser.

Acetaldehyde – found in perfume, dyes, fruit and fish preservatives, and flavor fragrances, which produce a fruity odor. It is a suspected animal carcinogen and has been classified in Group B2 as a probable human carcinogen of low carcinogenic hazard by the EPA. It can cause eye, skin and respiratory tract irritation. No information is available on the reproductive or developmental effects of acetaldehyde in humans; however, studies in animals have shown that acetaldehyde has crossed the placenta to the fetus.

Acetonitrile – found in perfume, dyes, and pharmaceuticals. It can cause irritation of the mucous membranes, weakness, headaches, tremor, numbness, and nausea. High concentrations can cause convulsions and **death**.

Benzyl chloride – found in perfume, dyes, pharmaceuticals, and a flavor fragrance. It was formerly used as an irritant gas in **chemical warfare**. It can cause skin, eye, lung, and mucous membrane irritation, dizziness, headache, fatigue, and is a suspected animal carcinogen. The EPA has classified benzyl chloride as a Group B2, which is a probable human carcinogen of low carcinogenic hazard.

Cinnamaldehyde – found in perfume and flavors. It can cause eye, nose, skin, and respiratory tract irritation.

Citronella – found in perfume, fabric softener, shampoo, and nail enamel remover. It can cause eye, nose, skin, and respiratory tract irritation.

Dimethyl sulfate – found in perfume, dyes, and pharmaceuticals. It was formerly used in **chemical warfare**. It is a suspected animal carcinogen and a Group B2, probable human carcinogen. It can cause eye, mouth, skin, and respiratory tract irritation. Severe exposure may cause lung, heart, kidney and central nervous system damage, convulsions, delirium, paralysis, coma, and even **death**.

Musk ambrette – found in perfume. It has been proven to cause central nervous system damage, weight loss and muscle weakness in laboratory animals.

Must tetralin (AETT) – was found in perfume, aftershave lotions, colognes and creams, and was used as a masking agent in unscented products. This chemical was found to cause irritability, degeneration of the brain neurons and changes in the spinal cord in laboratory animals. This chemical was voluntarily withdrawn by the fragrance industry in 1977, but it has not been banned by the FDA. It can be reintroduced into the fragrance industry at any time, and there are no guarantees that it is not being used now.

Styrene oxide – found in perfume and cosmetics. It can cause skin and eye irritation. In animals, it is known to be a central nervous system depressant.

Toluene (methyl benzene) – found in perfume, soap, cosmetics, nail polish removers, detergents, dyes, aerosol spray paints, paint strippers, spot removers, gasoline, antifreeze, and **explosives**. Petroleum crude oil is the largest source of toluene. It can cause damage to the lungs, liver, kidneys, heart, and central nervous system, skin and eye irritation, numbness, dizziness, tremors, headaches, confusion, unconsciousness, and **death**. Chronic exposure can cause loss of memory and muscle control, **brain damage**, problems with speech, hearing, and vision. Toluene was detected in **every** fragrance sample collected by the Environmental Protection Agency for a 1991 report. [13]

Synthetic Musk Linked to Environmental Risks

THE TOLEDO BLADE NEWS
By Michael Woods, Blade Science Editor
March 24, 1999

ANAHEIM, CA – Synthetic fragrances used in perfumes, soaps, detergents, fabric softeners, cosmetics, and scores of other consumer products have become a new and unexpected group of environmental contaminants, scientists said.

The chemicals are accumulating in human fat tissue, blood, breast milk, drinking water supplies, lakes and streams, fish and wildlife, and elsewhere in the environment, according to scientists interviewed here. They are presenting scientific reports at a national meeting of the American Chemical Society.

"I think there is reason for public concern about possible effects of these fragrances," said Dr. Sabastian Kevekordes of the University of Gottingen in Germany.

One compound, musk xylene, has carcinogenic, or cancer-causing, effects in laboratory mice, Dr. Kevekordes said. Another, musk ketone, damages genes in animal experiments and has other worrisome effects.

Many of the studies identifying synthetic musk compounds in human tissue and the environment have been done in Europe and Japan. Dr. Kevekordes said that synthetic musks are used just as widely, or more so, in the United States, where fragrances have been used even in trash bags and product packaging.

Dr. Gerhard G. Rimkus, another German expert interviewed at the meeting of scientists, estimated that 8,000 tons of synthetic musk fragrances are produced annually.

"Oh, absolutely they are used in the states," said Dr. Rimkus, who is with the Official Food and Veterinary Institute in Neumuenster. "Use is probably more extensive than in Europe or Japan. These are high-volume global chemicals. It's very hard to avoid them in consumer products."

Drs. Kevekordes and Rimkus said that American scientists generally are not as aware of the European findings. Dr. Rimkus said scientists and government regulators have lagged Europe and Japan in research on the synthetic musks.

Japan, he said, has banned musk xylene because of its ability to accumulate in fish and other aquatic life used as human food. Western European countries have agreed on a partial, voluntary phase-out of musk xylene, he said.

"On the basis of the precautionary principle, strong endeavors should be made by industry to move in the long term toward cessation of production and discharges of these synthetic musk compounds because of their poor degradability," Dr. Rimkus said.

"It must be possible to do without these substances," Dr. Kevekordes said. They are not essential chemicals, he said.

Dr. Kevekordes cited Dr. Herbert S. Rosenkranz, interim dean of the graduate school of public health at the University of Pittsburgh, as one of the American scientists most familiar with synthetic musks.

Dr. Rosenkranz said he is aware of the European research on musks, but has no direct knowledge of the findings and did not know of American scientists working intensively in the field.

Glenn Roberts, a spokesman for the Fragrance Manufacturers' Association in Washington, said he has not read the new studies. The association is a trade group representing companies that supply fragrance materials.

He said the studies seem to report information that is well-known to fragrance industry scientists.

"We're convinced as a result of a very extensive series of human health and environmental studies that there is no risk to human or the environment from these materials," Mr. Roberts said.

New studies in Canada have identified the same kind of environmental contamination with synthetic musks as detected in Europe, Dr. Rimkus said. He plans to do what may be the first independent tests of environment samples from the United States, and believes that contamination will be widespread.

Natural musk fragrances from the male deer, muskrats, a "musk beetle," and other animals are among the oldest ingredients in perfumes. The scarce, expensive natural musk extracts have been used in small amounts for thousands of years.

In the 20th century, chemists learned how to make synthetic compounds with a fragrance of musk. Use of musk fragrances skyrocketed, and the compounds are used in products that don't even have the odor of musk.

The compounds can be absorbed through the skin and tend to build up in fat tissue. They get into the environment in

GET A WHIFF OF THIS

sewage and wastewater. Dr. Rimkus said synthetic musk compounds are major chemical contaminants in many samples of water and fish.

Scientists know very little about the direct effects of synthetic musks, and even less about effects of the chemicals formed when musks eventually break down into other compounds. [14]

CHAPTER 4

ANDERSON LABORATORIES

SCIENTIFIC ARTICLE
(published in a peer-reviewed scientific journal)
Archives of Environmental Health

Acute Toxic Effects of Fragrance Products

Rosalind C. Anderson
Julius H. Anderson
Anderson Laboratories, Inc.
West Hartford, Vermont

ABSTRACT – To evaluate whether fragrance products can produce acute toxic effects in mammals, we allowed groups of male Swiss-Webster mice to breathe the emissions of five commercial colognes or toilet water for 1 h. We used the ASTM-E-981 test method to evaluate sensory irritation and pulmonary irritation.

We used a computerized version of this test to measure the duration of the break at the end of inspiration and the duration of the pause at the end of expiration.

Decreases in expiratory flow velocity indicated airflow limitation. We subjected the mice to a functional observational battery to probe for changes in nervous system function. The emissions of these fragrance products caused various combinations of sensory irritation, pulmonary irritation, decreases of expiratory airflow velocity, as well as alterations of the functional observational battery indicative of neurotoxicity. Neurotoxicity was more severe after mice were repeatedly exposed to the fragrance products. Evaluation of one of the test atmospheres with gas chromatography/mass spectrometry revealed the presence of chemicals for which irritant and neurotoxic properties had been documented previously. In summary, some fragrance products emitted chemicals that caused a variety of acute toxicities in mice.

FRAGRANCE PRODUCTS produce a pleasant odor via effects on the olfactory apparatus (first cranial nerve). Some individuals, however, report unpleasant reactions to fragrance products, 1,027 households sampled randomly in eastern North Carolina, 108 (10.5%) households reported that 1 or more individuals had adverse reactions to perfumes. Intolerance to fragrance products is also a frequent complaint of individuals who suffer multiple chemical sensitivity as a result of toxic exposure at the workplace and exposure to pesticides or remodeling, as well as individuals who suffer multiple chemical sensitivity of diverse etiologies.

In addition to our ability to sense odor, most mammals have another sense—the common chemical sense—mediated by the fifth cranial nerve. Stimulation of these receptors results in perception of irritancy or pungency; this process, called *sensory irritation* (SI), results in a local neurogenic inflammation. The ability of airborne molecules to cause this toxic event can be predicted quite accurately on the basis of their physical chemical parameters. Given that the typical fragrance product is a complex mixture of many volatile organic chemicals, it would not be surprising if some of the components of these mixtures might acutely effect the fifth cranial nerve endings (i.e., produce SI and neurogenic inflammation). In addition, one might expect some effects on the lower airways and/or absorption of some of these gases into the general circulation, and possibly some systemic or nervous system effects. [15]

Note: I would suggest your physician read the full text of this scientific article.

Requests for reprints can be sent to Rosalind C. Anderson, Ph.D., P.O. Box 123, West Hartford, VT 05084-0323.

ANDERSON LABORATORIES, INC.
West Hartford, Vermont

Toxic Effects of Air Freshener Emissions
Author(s): Anderson, Rosalind C.; Anderson, Julius H.

COMMERCIALLY MARKETED AIR FRESHENERS (AFs) would be valuable if they improved air quality and/or reduced health effects that result from air pollution. However, some individuals complain that some AFs are irritating, rather than beneficial. We know of no investigators who conducted studies to demonstrate an actual improvement of air quality from use of an AF, nor are we aware of any explorations of the potential adverse health effects of the emissions of these products.

In this study, we investigated one commercially available AF to evaluate whether the emissions contributed to poor indoor air quality and whether there were potentially harmful human health effects associated with exposure.

Conclusion
We can study some acute toxic effects of complex mixtures of chemicals (e.g., those offgassing from commercial AF). Although such studies do not allow us to assign toxicities to specific chemical components of the mixture, [19.20] the results are useful for screening; they demonstrate the need for further concern and research about the toxicity of the product tested. The emissions of this solid AF produced acute respiratory and neurotoxicity in mice, and they did not lower the toxic impact of the other pollutants tested. Collectively, toxicity data, chemical data, and MSDS information predict that some humans exposed to emissions of the AF we studied might experience some combination of eye, nose, and/or throat irritation; respiratory difficulty;

bronchoconstriction or an asthma-like reaction; and CNS reactions (e.g., dizziness, incoordination, confusion, fatigue). [16]

Submitted for publication July 23, 1996; revised; accepted for publication January 16, 1977. Requests for reprints should be sent to Julius H. Anderson, M.D., PhD., Anderson Laboratories, Inc., Box 323, West Hartford, VT 05084.

Note: I would suggest medical professionals obtain the full text of this scientific report.

CHAPTER 5

ABSTRACT

Abstract of Article on Dana Perfume Co.

TITLE: Health Hazard Evaluation Report HETA 91-026-2557, Dana Perfume Corporation, Mountaintop, Pennsylvania
AUTHORS: Y. Boudreau; L. Abrams; T Seitz.
INST. AUTHOR: National Inst. for Occupational Safety and Health, Cincinnati, OH, Hazard Evaluations and Technical Assistance Branch.

ABSTRACT: An investigation was begun regarding headaches, nausea, throat irritation, and tongue numbness occurring among employees in the "Spray Room" at the Dana Perfume Corporation (SIC-2844), Mountaintop, Pennsylvania, upon the request of management and Local 8-782 of the Oil, Chemical, and Atomic Workers International Union.
Twenty-six thousand bottles were filled on the average in one day at the facility. Area air samples and personal breathing zone revealed relatively low, but detectable, concentrations of volatile organic compounds, including ethanol (64175). Concentrations of beta-pinene (127913), p-cymeme (25155151), benzyl-acetate (140114), and limonene (138863) were also barely detectable.
The spray room's area air sample found no detectable levels of aldehydes. Although overexposures to perfume constituents were not found in this study, according to the authors, they concluded that **low** concentration exposures could cause some of the reported symptoms. The actuator placement area and the filling machine area were the most likely sources of the exposures, which were observed. The authors recommended that steps be taken to reduce the exposure levels in the spray room. [17]

CONNIE PITTS

CHAPTER 6

HALIFAX, NOVA SCOTIA OUTLAWS PERFUMES

THE REAL FACTS

Note from Nova Scotia: Perfume Stinks

Nova Scotia has outlawed perfume in public places since learning they contain toxic chemicals. The ban is observed in 80% of schools, in government buildings, and is expanding in private workplaces.

Anti-perfume activists who lobbied outside the City Hall in Halifax's capital, wearing gas masks, can consider this a victory. They complained that some of the chemicals in fragrances cause multiple chemical sensitivity, and 97% of fragrance chemicals are undisclosed.

The president of Citizens for a Safe Learning Environment, Karen Robinson, mentioned that this ban will affect the pocketbook of the fragrance industry. Considering the power of the fragrance industry, discrediting complaints only makes sense. People with MCS are not hypochondriacs, nor zealots.

An eighty-four-year-old lady, wearing a dab of perfume, was escorted out of a city council meeting at City Hall.

A seventeen-year-old pupil at Sheet Harbour High School almost got a criminal record in Canada, as he refused to give up his hair gel and deodorant. The teen was handed over to the Royal Canadian Mounted Police and was released without charge, but his teacher, sensitive to fragrance, blamed the scent for triggering a vomiting attack. She was backed by the school and referred to the incident as an assault. [18]

The "REAL" Facts the Fragrance Industry Doesn't Want You to Know

Betty Bridges visits Halifax

The following is a summary of the rebuttal to the fragrance industry's publicity campaign.

Halifax, Nova Scotia has been at the forefront when it comes to increasing awareness and educating people on the health issues related to fragranced products. The fragrance industry quickly enough realized that this was not an issue that was going to go away, and could very well spread to other areas, so they launched a publicity campaign to "discount" health concerns that have been raised.

The fragrance industry must appear sympathetic, while discounting the validity of those speaking out regarding the negative impact of fragrances. The industry came to Halifax to launch their campaign on June 20, 2000. The press was *not invited* to this conference. Instead, a press conference was scheduled for later that morning. The Scented Product Education and Information Association of Canada (SPEIAC), Scientific Advisory Committee of the Fragrance Materials Association, and Canadian Cosmetic, Toiletry, and Fragrance Association (CCTFA), sponsored an educational forum in which representatives from Health Canada, individuals representing the anti-scent movement, and Halifax policy makers were invited.

Charles Low of the CCTFA moderated the meeting. Of course, the industry contends that there is no "scientific" basis for fragrance bans. There was an opportunity for questions to be asked "after" the presentation but no opportunity for advocates of scent-reduction policies to present the extensive scientific data available.

A point-by-point examination of the materials presented and questions raised by the industry's press release and ad follows. The public has a right to know more than "tidbits" in order to form opinions and make decisions affecting their health.

Response to SPEIAC Press Release and Ad Campaign

Assertion 1:
Carl Carter, SPEIAC Communication Director, suggested that it was time to get the facts straight regarding claims being made by scent ban advocates and mentioned that the scent free policies in Halifax appeared to be based on lack of factual information.

Reply:
Fragrances are respiratory irritants, which can trigger asthma as well as other respiratory problems, allergies, migraines, and other neurological adverse effects. Small amounts can trigger symptoms in people who suffer these effects. Fragrances add to air pollution, as they are volatile compounds. Additionally, there are environmental concerns with synthetic musk compounds being found in waterways and aquatic wildlife throughout the world. These facts are well documented in peer-reviewed scientific journals.

Assertion 2:
Carter continued to acknowledge that they respect the fact that some individuals may react to many common everyday substances, including fragrances, but at the same time, he claims that scented products are as safe as the foods we eat and the many other products we use daily.

Reply:
Very often, the news media reports incidents of food poisonings and other concerns related to food safety. Flavors in foods, for example, are often the same chemicals used in scented products, so concerns are valid.

Assertion 3:
Carter said that accurate information and the best available accepted science should be based on responsible public policy-making. He also claimed that, that is why SPEIAC is making an effort to correct the misinformation being circulated.

Reply:
Those with asthma, vasomotor rhinitis, and migraines must avoid exposures to triggers. Because labeling does not allow one to determine which chemicals are problematic, and there are no tests to determine exactly which fragrance chemicals are the trigger, limiting or eliminating personal care scented products is not sufficient to prevent problems. One can only avoid ALL fragranced products as a means of preventing triggers.

Assertion 4:
Bill Troy, Chair of the Scientific Advisory Committee of the Fragrance Materials Association (FMA), said that fragrance industry associations around the world work closely with the Research Institute for Fragrance Materials (RIFM), and that this is a responsible industry that takes *safety* seriously.

Reply:
Out of 3,000 raw fragrance materials in use, the RIFM has evaluated less than half. Chemical combinations often act very different from singular materials, in combinations, as they involve additive, modifying, and synergetic effects.

Testing is not routinely done for neurological, respiratory, or systemic effects, as testing by the RIFM focuses on acute and oral toxicity and skin effects.

Bill Troy, Ph.D. was working at AVON in 1975 while, during routine animal patch skin testing, something was discovered in the product that was turning the skin of the animals blue. Acetylethyletramethyletralin (AETT) was found to cause serious neurological conditions and discoloration of the skin and organs of animals, also penetrating the skin, further tests revealed. Had there not been a change in skin color, the neurotoxicity of this chemical may not ever have been discovered.

AVON was the only company that used AETT whose testing discovered it posed serious health risks.

For over twenty years, AETT had been in common use when this discovery was made in 1975. No company, including the company originally using the material, had discovered that it was *severely* neurotoxic. Although voluntarily withdrawn from use in 1977, there were no recalls or public notifications of products on the shelf.

Generally, the RIFM doesn't evaluate raw materials for safety until the patent expires. Materials can be used in common use for close to twenty years before any evaluation may occur outside of the company producing them.

Over the last few decades, much information has been learned. Many materials once considered safe are now found to be unsafe. More information regarding toxicity and danger is available now than (it was) over a decade ago—not only of singular chemicals but of combinations. Therefore, much more aggressive evaluation is vital and necessary. Respiratory, neurological, and systemic testing is needed. To contend that "there is no proof our products are not safe" is hardly the attitude expected from a self-regulated industry. If the industry wants to continue to self-regulate and avoid increasing regulation, it must leave no doubt that the products are safe for the user, those inadvertently exposed, and the environment.

Assertion 5:
For hundreds of years, fragrances have been composed of grain alcohol and water—with the same type of purity we drink in beverages—together with essential oils.

Reply:
Perfumes are typically considered the most concentrated form of a scented product, with 10–30 percent fragrance and the remainder consisting of ethyl alcohol. The number one cause of allergic reactions to laundry products and cosmetics is fragrance, despite relatively low concentrations.

The percentage of alcohol to the percentage of fragrance is the only basic composition that has remained mostly unchanged. However, the "fragrance" portion of these products is *considerably different* from what it was nearly thirty years ago. New formulations are made of primarily synthetic fragrance oils, not essential oils from plants. When the applications for these materials are different and newer materials are used, history of use does not apply.

Assertion 6:
Carter stated that ingredients in scented products are safety tested, and they do not contain the dangerous substances that some people are claiming . . . .

Reply:
Reputable scientific data and Material Safety Data Sheets raises concerns about the safety of materials used in fragrances. Some ingredients have not been tested at all, and others have not been tested adequately. It is up to the industry to provide peer-reviewed evaluations of the materials, if this information is not accurate. Unless this should happen, the scientific data available must be used.

Assertion 7:
People also need to know that a synthetic material doesn't mean it is harmful. Safety of a substance is not determined by natural origin or if it is synthetic. Synthetic materials often help us preserve natural sources and are often purer.

Reply:
A natural material is not always safer than a synthetic material; however, natural materials have a much longer history of use, so more is known about them. The history of use argument to modern fragrance formulations is something the fragrance industry often tries to apply. When either materials or use is different, history of use does not apply. Natural materials, although safely used for centuries, became problematic when used in different applications.

Assertion 8:
Health Canada regulates perfumes and personal care products.

Reply:
Testing products prior to marketing is not required. Fragrance ingredients of the product do not have to be revealed to any regulatory agency. Even minimal regulation is rarely enforced. Canadian law does require warning of known health hazards. Fragrances are known to be respiratory irritants and skin sensitizers.

GET A WHIFF OF THIS

Despite these established health hazards, products do not bear a warning.

Assertion 9:
Carter added that public policy should be based on accurate information and not beliefs, which are vital to protecting individual rights and freedoms. He referred to the widespread and public policies in the region as erroneous beliefs.

Reply:
Different positions on the safety of fragrance products are obviously vastly different. A high cooperative effort would be the best way to resolve these differences. People who suffer adverse reactions to fragrances can provide valuable information to the industry that could help pinpoint unsafe or problematic materials so they can be eliminated from use. Awareness and consideration of those who suffer adverse effects from fragrances could be increased by education. Problems will only increase—not go away. Whether the battle lines are drawn or the problem is resolved will be up to the industry.

Assertion 10:
SPEIAC continues to support responsible use of scented products, advising that everyone has a personal scent "circle" about an arm's length from the body. Exercising restraint when using scented products so that is not detectable outside your scent circle is what the Association recommends.

Reply:
Keeping a scent within a "personal" scent circle is virtually impossible. Such a suggestion ignores basic scientific principles. Diffusion of a material in the air involves many factors. It is impossible to control these factors in conditions of actual use. Once in the air, containment is impossible. Some of each fragranced product used is left behind in the air wherever the user goes. They can't take their "circle" of air with them.

There is always a background of "fragrance" in the air, due to the widespread use of fragranced products both in personal and environmental applications. Considering only singular products certainly does not adequately address the problems. Scented laundry products, air fresheners, cleaners, toiletries, and perfumes used primarily for "scent" must be taken into consideration.

Many fragrance products diffuse into the air quickly and can be detected before even encountering the person wearing them—and long after that person has left, as many fragranced products are formulated deliberately to be high impact.

The industry is advocating what they consider a solution to something that they should know will never work. [19]

CHAPTER 7

SCENTED CANDLES –
THE REAL DIRT

GET A WHIFF OF THIS

Dangers of Fragranced Candles

ENVIRONMENTAL ILLNESS SOCIETY OF CANADA (EISC)
536 Dovercourt Avenue,
Ottawa, ON K2A OT9 Canada

With the current popularity of scented and aromatic candles, the following information is pertinent to consumers, as they NEED to be aware for the health and safety of their families.

Burning candles can expose your children to lead emissions.

There is a commonly used and very popular consumer product that presents some serious concerns regarding toxic exposures to children. In the last few years, scented and aromatic candles have experienced unprecedented sales. Due to the increasing use of scented candles in the home, effects of their emissions have drawn the attention of Indoor Air Experts, Environmental Health Professionals, the Consumer Product Safety Commission, and Toxicologists.

Candles can expose children to lead.

Lead core wicks are still being used by some candle makers. This is particularly worrisome, as infants, small children, and their mothers (especially pregnant women), are exposed quite often, since they are the ones who spend a great deal of time inside the home.

What other toxic ingredients are in some scented candles?

In addition to lead, candles can also present long term exposures to the following:

Acetone	Carbon Monoxide	Tetrachloroethene
Benzene	Cyclopentene	Toluene
2-Butanone	Ethylbenzene	1,1,1-Trichloroethane

Carbon Disulfide	Lead	Trichloroethene
Carbon Tetrachloride	Mercury	Trichlorofluoromethane
Cresol	Phenol	Xylene
Chlorobenzene	Styrene	

Air chamber tests of candles detected and measured these compounds. Average particle size is .06 microns. The last round of testing indicated the release of **DIETHYL PHTHALATE**. It was discovered that the candles off-gass **BENZENE** without being lit.

Candle manufacturers are not accountable to anyone—not even consumers.

Ingredients are not listed because candle makers don't have to list them. Manufacturers and retailers of candles are not compelled to disclose toxic, hazardous, or carcinogenic compounds used in their products or an ingredient list at all. There are absolutely no regulations pertaining to this consumer product, according to the Federal Trade Commission (FTC) and the Consumer Products Safety Commission (CPSC).

Candle emissions raise a number of concerns and issues, such as:

- the indoor air quality of homes, especially where infants and young children reside
- Black Soot Deposition (BSD) in homes, as this destroys the contents of a home, as well as the ventilation system
- toxic compound emissions
- particle matter lead exposures to consumers
- the lack of government regarding the expanding candle industry

The candle industries have made false and absurd claims and statements regarding Aromatherapy and their effects on health and well being . . . .

It's crucial that consumers become aware of possible toxic exposures to respirable particles from candle emissions. The particles in the emissions average .06 microns in size. Forty to fifty percent of ingested toxins are absorbed, whereas 100% of respirable particles

GET A WHIFF OF THIS

this small are absorbed. Parents must have access to this information if they are to protect their infants and toddlers. Young children tend to move around more on carpeting, placing their faces close to the source and inhaling some of these particles.

According to a toxicologist, candle emissions may indeed pose a significantly higher risk of health effects not only from lead but also from VOCs, solvents, and PAHs (Polycyclic Aromatic Hydrocarbons). Children's respiration rate is faster than most adults. Children are more active, increasing respiration even more. A child has a tendency to breathe more through the mouth than an adult, and the ratio of toxins to body mass is higher, due to their smaller size and weight. Certain toxins, solvents, and heavy metals are stored in body fat, bones, and organs, and evidence of exposure may not manifest itself until many years later or when the body is stressed, such as periods of rapid growth, puberty, illness, and pregnancy. Some of the compounds in candle emissions are actually capable of damaging or mutating DNA. Any steps you can take to minimize exposures would be wise, as children are especially vulnerable to toxic exposures. [20]

Candles, Toxic Emissions, and Property Damage

The following is a summary of information provided by Cathy Flanders, who has been at the forefront of addressing health and safety issues involving candles.

Pregnant women and children should avoid Toxic Emissions from candles.

With the current "candle-craze" and increased candle burning in homes, expectant mothers need to be aware of the emissions from candles that are toxic, reproductive toxins, neurotoxins, and/or carcinogenic. This has become a growing concern for the EPA and children's health agencies. Recently, funding has been appropriated from the National Institute of Health to test and evaluate levels of emissions from "scented" candles. Levels of toxic VOC & PAH (Polycyclic Aromatic Hydrocarbon) compounds can rise quickly inside a home to a level that poses a danger to you and your unborn baby simply from burning a few candles at a time. Some candles contain substantial quantities of lead in the wicks, which release fine particles that can be inhaled because of their minute size. The fine particles are absorbed into the bloodstream, exposing you and your baby to very harmful cumulative toxin. If you feel you cannot refrain from candle burning, 100% beeswax candles are free of synthetic ingredients.

Gel Candles contain plasticizers and phthalates—extremely toxic, especially to children. You may wonder how they can sell it. There are no laws or standards governing the manufacture of candles. They can put whatever they want into candles and not label it.

A lawsuit was filed recently against a very popular retailer, which had lead in their candles, leaving a home contaminated with lead dust after months of using this particular brand. Particles from candles are attracted to synthetic fibers, such as carpet. Do you place your baby on the floor to play?

Hundreds of homeowners around the country have reported substantial property damage to their home's interiors, and contents, due to candle soot deposits on everything from ceilings, walls, carpet, toys, computers, and other electronics, as well as plastics.

There are a few things that are important to do as soon as possible if you have damage of substantial monetary value:

1. Try to recall a time frame, to the best of your ability, when the candles that are suspected of causing the damage were burned. Try to answer the following questions:

    How often were they burned?
    How many were burned, and how many at a time?
    Where were they located when you burned them?

Also, you may want to have receipts for your candle purchases. Collect all relevant information into a file so facts will be consistent, and make notes with contact names and what they had to say.

2. Contact your Homeowners Insurance Company and/or Agent.

3. Contact the candle retailer and manufacturer and get your report of damage as a result of product use "on the record."

4. File an incident report with the Consumer Product Safety Commission (CPSC).
    Their toll-free number is: 1-800-638-2772.

Some recent developments:

* A front page *Wall Street Journal* article on 3/31/99 reported on this very issue of candle soot damage to homes.

* An ASTM Sub-Committee was formed in cooperation with the CPSC to examine candle performance with sooting being one of the many issues on the table.

* A presentation was made at the largest IAQ (Indoor Air Quality) Conference last month dealing solely with the issue of soot deposition & health hazards from candle emissions.

* There was a technical meeting this year at the NCA meeting to discuss candle emissions.

* Over 25 candle makers, manufacturers, suppliers, and retailers have had Proposition 65 notices filed against them for toxic or hazardous ingredients without warning or disclosure.

* A Class Action is awaiting certification against a worldwide retailer of candles which contained lead.

* A number of civil cases have been initiated across the country by homeowners in an attempt to recover the expense of damage they incurred due to candle use. [21]

CHAPTER 8

THE EFFECTS OF CHEMICALS ON WOMEN AND CHILDREN

MONEY RULES

Chemicals Pose a Higher Risk for Females

The following is a summary from Pamela Smarr's writing.

Many women and girls have become walking toxic dumps. Females are at a higher risk considering the fact that many toxic chemicals are fat-soluble, therefore storing in body fat. Women and girls have a higher percentage of body fat.

Several toxins interfere with proper function of the hormone system, which can affect a woman's ability to reproduce. Toxins, which act as endocrine disrupters, can affect the genetic make-up of offspring. Some toxins can hurt the developing fetus, since they pass from the mother's placenta.

We are using children like canaries in the mine, warns Dr. Phillip Landigran, a pediatrician who helps lead the children's health initiative of the U.S. Environmental Protection Agency. Out of more then 75,000 chemicals used in the U.S., only a small percentage of them have ever been tested for their cancer causing potential.

The EPA began to put in place a process for determining which chemicals are endocrine disrupters this year. Congress is being fought by large companies obviously worried about reactions from consumers, so this work has not been fully funded by Congress.

Dr. Landigran warns that since World War II, with the widespread use of untested petroleum-based chemicals, we have been conducting medical experiments on generations, both current and future.

After heart disease, cancer is the second leading cause of death in the U.S. Cancer is the fourth leading cause of death in children. This enormous increase cannot be attributed to genetic changes, as the increases are much too rapid between generations. There seems to be an environmental connection, as of the 6 million people worldwide diagnosed in 1996 with cancer, 3.8 million were living in developing countries. In the U.S., genetic risk factors for breast cancer are approximately 10%.

Cancers that have increased with the most alarming trends are brain, breast, liver, kidney, prostate, esophagus, melanoma, bone marrow, and non-Hodgkin's lymphoma. The number of people with non-Hodgkin's lymphoma has tripled since 1950.

How many people in your church, neighborhood, or workplace do you hear about with breast cancer or prostate cancer? How many children with cancer? Many cancers have roots caused from environmental damage.

Asthma has increased 40% in children since 1980. It has become the leading reason for hospitalization of children, as well as the leading cause of missing school.

Acute leukemia has risen 10% in children under fourteen and brain tumors have increased 30%. Children develop leukemia three to nine times more often when pesticides are used around their homes.

As a society, we may be poisoning ourselves to the point of death. Scientific evidence points to environmental contamination as a major factor for the increase of cancer.

Other chronic conditions, such as asthma, immune system dysfunction, thyroid malfunctioning, premature puberty in girls, unsafe blood glucose levels, and endometriosis are being linked to environmental contamination.

How much longer are we willing to pay the price in terms of women and children's lives? [22]

GET A WHIFF OF THIS

Environmental Research Foundation

MONEY RULES

The following is a summary from Rachel's Environment & Health Weekly #680
- December 16, 1999 -

One of the most important trends of the last half of the twentieth century was the spread of democracy into many countries that had never enjoyed it before. At the same time, democracy within the U.S. continued to shrivel as the wealthy elite gained increasing control. All three branches of government actively encouraged this shift of power from "the rest of us" to the wealthy.

In April, the U.S. Supreme Court made it easier for the wealthy to curry favor with government officials. The court ruled that substantial gifts to a government official are legal unless the official performs a "specific official act" in return for a gift. The matter came before the court because Sun-Diamond Growers of California gave gifts worth $5,900 to Mike Espy when he was Secretary of Agriculture. Since Espy did not perform any specific official act on behalf of Sun-Diamond in return for the gifts, the gifts were legal, the court ruled. The American League of Lobbyists expressed relief at the court's ruling. Lobbyists now know that they can shower Congress with gifts without running afoul of the law. One favorite tactic is to give money to Congressional staffers, rather than directly to members of Congress. Another favorite is to pay for lavish vacations for members of Congress, disguised as "fact-finding trips."

By November, it was clear that the Supreme Court's April ruling would deepen the level of corruption in Congress. Federal prosecutors dropped almost all charges against Ann Eppard, former legislative chief of staff for Congressman Bud Shuster, a Republican from Pennsylvania. Between 1989 and 1993, while she was Schuster's chief of staff, Ms. Eppard accepted $230,000 in gifts from a lobbyist. She was subsequently indicted on seven counts. In November, she pleaded guilty to one misdemeanor charge for taking illegal compensation and agreed to pay a fine of $5,000. The other six charges were dropped. Federal prosecutors defended their plea bargain saying the Supreme Court ruling made it impossible to expect a conviction. Ms. Eppard now runs her own lobbying firm, Ann Eppard Associates.

On December 5, *The New York Times* reported that state governors' offices are now thoroughly soaked in money, just as federal offices have been for more than a decade. "The 'permanent campaign' that has become a fixture of races for the presidency and the Senate has now descended upon the 50 state capitols," the *Times* reported.

With the wealthy legally empowered to pour money into government, one might expect the government to return the favor. Late in 1999, *The New York Times* reported that ". . . the Internal Revenue Service [the nation's tax collection agency] is reducing its efforts to find cheating by businesses and high-income individuals, and stepping up investigations into two forms of cheating that are more likely to involve the working poor than the affluent."

Since 1995, the poorest 20% of families have seen their annual incomes reduced by $577, falling to $8,047 annually. The situation was worse for the poorest 10% who lost $814 per year. Children were hardest hit. In 1995, 88% of poor children were helped by food stamps. By 1998, only 70% of poor children were being helped. "There are people at the bottom who are worse off," said Ron Haskins, staff director of the Congressional subcommittee that wrote the "welfare reform" law. "We need to do something about that," he said in August, but by December, nothing had been done.

Meanwhile, 20% of American households have more debt than assets—which is to say, they have a negative net worth. In early 1999, thirty-five million Americans were living in poverty.

The number of poor people would be considerably larger if prisoners were counted. Two-thirds of prisoners are serving sentences for non-violent offenses. America's federal "drug czar," General Barry McCaffrey, refers to the U.S. prison system as "America's Internal gulag." [23]

CHAPTER 9

C.T.F.A.

Cosmetic, Toiletry, and Fragrance Association

The leading U.S. trade association for personal care products industry is the Cosmetic, Toiletry, and Fragrance Association[*], with more than 500 member companies. The CTFA works to protect the freedom of the industry to compete in responsible and fair marketplace. The CTFA also represents lobbying efforts in state governments and Congress. It represents the cosmetic industry in issues that involve the EPA, FDA, and other government agencies.

In 1976, the CTFA established the Cosmetic Ingredients Review Board (CIR). The purpose of the CIR is to review the safety of cosmetic materials. The CIR does not review ingredients of fragrance. The Research Institute for Fragrance Materials (RIFM) gathers data regarding the safety of fragrance ingredients. The International Fragrance Association (IFRA) then reviews the information and formulates guidelines for use.

Contact Information

Cosmetic, Toiletry, and Fragrance Association
1100 17th Street, N.W., Suite 300
Washington, DC 20036
Phone: 202-331-1770
Fax: 202-331-1969

Cosmetic Ingredients Review
1101 17th Street, N.W. Suite 310
Washington, DC 20036-4702
Phone: 202-331-0651
Fax: 202-331-1969

---

[*] http://www.ctfa.org/

CHAPTER 10

GOVERNMENT KNOWLEDGE

GET A WHIFF OF THIS

Safe Notification Information for Fragrances
[SNIFF]

Bill Status & Summary

This information is current as of 7/28/01.

Bill Summary & Status for the 107th Congress

H.R. 1947
Sponsor: Rep. Schakowsky, Janice D. (Introduced 5/22/2001)
Latest Major Action: 6/1/2001 Referred to House Subcommittee
Title: To amend the Federal Food, Drug, and Cosmetic Act to require that fragrances containing known toxic substances or allergens be labeled accordingly.

TITLE(S): (Italics indicate a title for a portion of a bill)

SHORT TITLE(S) AS INTRODUCED:
Safe Notification and Information for Fragrances Act

OFFICIAL TITLE AS INTRODUCED:
To amend the Federal Food, Drug, and Cosmetic Act to require that fragrances containing known toxic substances or allergens be labeled accordingly.

STATUS:

5/22/2001:
Referred to the House Committee on Energy and Commerce
6/1/2001:
Referred to the Subcommittee on Health

COMMITTEE(S):

Connie Pitts

Committee/Subcommittee
Activity:
House Energy and Commerce
Referral

Subcommittee on Health
Referral

RELATED BILL DETAILS:

NONE

AMENDMENT(S):

NONE

COSPONSORS(2), ALPHABETICAL [followed by Cosponsors withdrawn]: (Sort : by date)

Rep Berkley, Shelley – 5-22-2001
Rep Fattah, Chaka – 7/18/2001

SUMMARY AS OF:
5/22/2001 – Introduced

Safe Notification and Information for Fragrances Act – Amends the Federal Food, Drug, and Cosmetic Act to label a cosmetic as misbranded if it is a fragrance that contains a known toxic substance or allergen unless it bears a label stating the fact and the common or usual name of such substance or allergen. [9]

GET A WHIFF OF THIS

Federal Aviation Administration (FAA)

FAA Proposes Fine Against Bath & Body Works For Hazardous Materials Violations.
Dec. 19, 1997

WASHINGTON – The Federal Aviation Administration (FAA) has proposed fining Bath & Body Works of Columbus, Ohio a $750,000 civil penalty for shipping improperly packaged hazardous materials.

In FAA's notice of proposed penalty issued Dec. 3, Bath & Body Works, which operates a chain of retail cosmetic stores, is cited for knowingly offering hazardous materials for transportation by air when the materials were not properly packaged and in the condition for shipment required by the Department of Transportation (DOT) hazardous materials regulations.

In October 1994, the company applied for and was granted an exemption for the shipment of ethyl alcohol-based cosmetics as consumer commodities. These ethyl alcohol-based cosmetics are regulated materials that have flash points of less than 100 degrees Fahrenheit. Under the exemption, Bath & Body Works was still required to meet the DOT regulations for packaging and quantity limitations.

On at least 23 separate occasions between Dec. 12, 1995, and Jan. 31, 1996, Bath & Body Works offered Federal Express Corp. shipments of these hazardous materials that did not comply with the terms of exemption in that they either exceeded quantity limitations or were improperly packaged. These violations were discovered because each of the 23 shipments leaked.

In its notice to Bath & Body Works, FAA stated that it is proposing a $750,000 fine. The company has 30 days from the receipt of FAA's letter to respond to the notice.

An electronic version of this news release is available via the World Wide Web at: http://www.faa.gov/[*]

---

[*] Note: Presently available at: http://www1.faa.gov/apa/pr16597.htm

GET A WHIFF OF THIS

Governor Bush's Proclamation
Declaring May 7–13, 2000
"MCS Awareness Week"
in the state of Florida

To learn if your state's governor supports MCS Awareness Week in May, please read:

http://www.rtk.net.ncci/NCCIMCSAwareness.htm

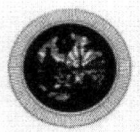

Jeb Bush
Governor of the State of Florida

Multiple Chemical Sensitivity Week

WHEREAS, Multiple Chemical Sensitivity (MCS) is a chronic condition for which there is no known cure; and

WHEREAS, MCS symptoms include chronic fatigue, muscle and joint pain, rashes, asthma, short-term memory loss, headaches and other respiratory and neurological problems; and

WHEREAS, MCS is recognized by the Americans with Disabilities Act, the Social Security Administration, U.S. Housing and Urban Development, U.S. Environmental Protection Agency and other governmental agencies and commissions;

NOW, THEREFORE, I, Jeb Bush, Governor of the state of Florida, do hereby extend greetings and best wishes to all observing *Multiple Chemical Sensitivity Week*, May 7-13, 2002.

IN WITNESS WHEREOF, I have hereunto set my hand and caused the Great Seal of the state of Florida to be affixed at Tallahassee, the Capital, this 1st day of March in the year of our Lord two thousand two.

GOVERNOR

---

* This document was obtained from: http://www.ourlittleplace.com.

GET A WHIFF OF THIS

To Report Adverse Health Effects of Fragrances Whether to Yourself or a Family Member, Contact:

Mr. Lark Lambert (mailto:LZL@cfsan.fda.gov)
HFS FDA
Office of Cosmetics and Colors
Cosmetic Adverse Reaction Monitoring Program
200 C St. SW
Washington, DC 20204
Phone: 202/418-3182

You may also wish to contact your government representatives. If you do not have access to a computer, you may call your State Capitol Building for a list of your representatives.

Government Links can be found online, below:

http://www.senate.gov

http://www.house.gov

DISABLING EFFECTS FROM SYNTHETIC FRAGRANCES, WHICH WOULD INCLUDE DEATH, ARE CONSIDERED A LOW PRIORITY WITH THE FDA, ACCORDING TO AN FDA SPOKESPERSON CONTACTED BY BETTY BRIDGES.

What the U.S. Government [FDA] Is Doing About It

GET A WHIFF OF THIS

CHAPTER 11

WEBSITES
SAFER PRODUCTS

Informative Websites:

http://www.fpinva.org/
Owned by Betty Bridges, RN,
Head of the Fragranced Products Information Network

http://www.ehnca.org/
Owned by Barbara Wilke,
Environmental Health Network of California

http://www.cancerresearchamerica.org/cosmetics.html
Owned by James W. Coleman, Ph.D.,
President/CEO
Cancer Research Center of America, Inc.

http://www.andersonlaboratories.com/
Owned by Drs. Julius and Rosalind Anderson,
Anderson Laboratories, Inc.

http://www.nottoopretty.org/
Owned by Coming Clean,
The Environmental Working Group,
Health Care Without Harm, and
Women's Voices of the Earth
(regarding phthalates)

Safer Products

Since many alleged "organic" products are not always organic, or may be volatile, I will mention a few products that I use and personally consider safer. Many products claiming to be perfume and dye-free are often loaded with perfume. I found this to be true of a grocery store's off-brand laundry detergent. It was heavily scented, and I have called the manufacturer to voice my complaint.

If one feels that they simply *must* have some kind of fragrance, "pure" essential oils may be a better alternative than synthetic fragrances. It is also important to use them with caution, as they may be sensitizing to the skin. Using too much could be harmful. More can be learned about pure essential oils on Betty Bridge's website.

Lotions:
Personally, I use Aveeno Fragrance-Free lotion for my skin, including my hands. Lubriderm also makes a fragrance-free lotion. Vaseline Intensive Care Fragrance-Free lotion is not truly fragrance-free.

I have found fragrance-free suntan lotions. I use Neutrogena Sensitive Skin, SPF 30, free of irritating chemicals, or Banana Boat. Simply look for products without the word fragrance or perfume. Adult fragrance-free sunscreen lotions may be fine for children. I have not found a fragrance-free suntan lotion made specifically for children, without shopping for expensive products online.

I use Complex 15 (Schering-Plough) for my face, and it is fragrance-free. This product is available at Walgreens or Rite-Aid. Oil of Olay may still have a fragrance-free face cream, but I purchased it, once, and something in it gave my skin a burning sensation.

Edge makes a fragrance-free shaving foam. Aftershaves are pointless. A splash of cold water will work just as well.

Deodorants:
Arm & Hammer Unscented anti-perspirant & deodorant is actually unscented.

Almay sells a fragrance-free, Clear Gel anti-perspirant & deodorant.

Shampoo and Conditioner:
Fragrance-free shampoos and conditioners are nearly impossible to find in grocery stores. Beware of many alleged herbal shampoos at health food stores as well. Many products are not what they claim to be. Neutrogena makes one fragrance-free dandruff shampoo, which is T/Sal. Look for the red box, and be certain to read the label. I have found some fragrance-free shampoos and conditioners at Wild Oats. One brand is Pure Essentials. Be careful, as they make more than one line of fragrance-free shampoo and conditioners. One is actually free, and the other is not.

Aveda has a fragrance-free shampoo and conditioner. Be sure to read labels, as many of their products do contain the word fragrance.

Hair gels are difficult to find, fragrance-free, but some health food stores *do* have them.

Hairspray:
I have yet to find a "safe" hair spray. Mixing lukewarm water with sugar, and shaking well, may do the trick.

Magick Botanicals sells a fragrance-free hair spray, which could be safer. Magick Botanicals can be ordered through NEEDS (website and number listed near end of page).

Clinique sells an unscented, non-aerosol hair spray, but again, I'm not certain about the ingredients listed. The ingredients do not include ethanol, butane, or fragrance.

Nail polish:
I do not wear nail polish but recently learned that Almay sells a line of nail polish, claiming it does not contain toluene or formaldehyde.

Soap:
I've purchased Dove fragrance-free soap, but I have heard complaints from some people regarding this soap. Dove's *Unscented* bar soap is highly fragranced. There are other fragrance-free soaps, but people must simply shop around. Some soaps and body washes can be found at Wild Oats or other health food stores.

For laundry:
I use Seventh Generation or OxiClean. Borax is another safer product. Some health food stores sell safer stain remover products. Seventh Generation also makes a fabric softener. Be sure to read the list of ingredients.

For tubs and sinks:
I use BonAmi. Nothing else is needed.
   Vinegar can clean and also kill bacteria. The smell might not be pleasant to some people, but it is a safer alternative, as is baking soda.
   For dusting, I use Swiffer cloths (dry only).
   I have also found many safer products at health food stores, including dishwasher detergent, dishwashing liquids, and mirror, window, and glass cleaners.

Furniture polish:
HOPE'S Premium Wood Care is solvent free, non-toxic, zero VOC, non-flammable, contains no chemical odor, and moisturizes wood.

Make-up:
I have found many fragrance-free make-ups, including lipsticks. Almay is fragrance-free. Clinique sells fragrance-free make-up and face care products. Cover Girl sells a fragrance-free foundation. One must shop carefully and read labels.

Air fresheners:
I am not aware of any safe air fresheners. Opening a window is the best advice I can offer.

I do believe, in the future, we will see a higher demand for more fragrance-free and non-toxic products hit the market. Eventually, it may be inevitable.
   Many hard to find *safer* products can be found at:

The Living Source
(254) 776-4878 or their 24 hr. voice order: 1-800-662-8787
http://www.livingsource.com/

GET A WHIFF OF THIS

Eco-Products
3655 Frontier Ave.
Boulder, CO 80301
http://www.ecoproducts.com/

NEEDS
http://www.needs.com/
1-800-634-1380

Disclaimer: *I am not suggesting what products may or may not be used, nor endorsing products I've listed. Some products, listed above, may bother some people, especially those with MCS.*

CONCLUSION

Despite a report to our government (99th Congress) from the National Academy of Sciences in 1986, suggesting fragrances be tested for neurotoxicity; despite the efforts of one Congresswomen, Janice Schakowsky, who introduced the SNIFF Act, (Safe Notification Information for Fragrances) Bill HR 1947; and despite a legal petition filed against a popular perfume to the FDA, has the FDA addressed this serious health issue?

Smoking has been banned in most public buildings. If the purpose of banning tobacco smoke is to reduce carcinogens in the air, then I believe we have failed, unless fragrance chemicals are also banned. Synthetic fragrances are an intrusive invasion of shared breathing space. It's time to rid the air of overpowering perfumes, colognes, and other scented products in public buildings. It would be a refreshing change to dine in a restaurant without overpowering chemicals dominating the aroma of food. It would be nice to go *anywhere* without being assaulted with these chemicals. Going to a medical facility, without breathing neurotoxins and carcinogens, would be a great start in the right direction.

Many men wear fragrances, as well as women and pre-teens. The industry is currently expanding its market. Children as young as three are targeted for "kid" versions of adult products. Some fragrance companies make "baby" colognes and aromatherapy products for children and infants. Many famous celebrities often have their names affiliated with fragrances, such as Elizabeth Taylor, Celine Dion, and Jennifer Lopez (J.Lo). Do I believe they know the contents of the products they endorse? Personally, I doubt that they know.

Perfumes, in centuries past, were used for the purpose of masking body odor, specifically for people who didn't bathe. Today, most Americans shower on a daily basis yet continue to drench themselves with hazardous substances with the misconception that they are safe products. Clever advertising, on behalf of the fragrance industry, has convinced many people that clothes must smell fresh for days and that houses must have the "smell" of clean—all at the expense of human health.

Since many people will probably continue to desire fragrances, one would think the fragrance industries could make them safe, or at least safer. Today's synthetic fragrances are not made responsibly, and therefore, people cannot be expected to wear them responsibly. Today's fragrances cannot be expected to stay at an arm's length when the chemicals quickly become airborne.

Some perfume *names* sound like dead giveaways to me, such as POISON or OPIUM. Other perfume names sound as if they are targeting our youth, such as perfumes ending in the word Homme. I think the name Mambo may have appeal to the Latino population, for example. There are numerous perfume names, some of which sound contradictory, and others that simply have initials or numbers rather than names. The fragrance industry is likely to target anyone who is apt to buy their products.

Who knows how many people *may* have died as a result of toxic perfume poisoning, since coroner reports, or death certificates, may only confirm cause of death as asthma, crib death, or cancer yet never know the source. We will never know.

It is evident that many women are getting breast cancer—and at younger ages. No one is immune to the harmful effects of these ubiquitous chemicals, which are now in most personal care products. Asthma has also become the "norm." This should not be considered acceptable.

What the fragrance industry has done, in my opinion, is no different from what the tobacco industries have done for years. Many additives, which tobacco companies were sued for, are fragrance chemicals. [24] Knowledge is the key, and now you hold the key.

The fragrance industry does not want safety and health effects to become public knowledge. That could hurt business. Discounting aspects of MCS is one of the deliberate actions taken by the fragrance industry. In addition to concerns regarding asthma, migraines, and sinus problems, the accumulation of fragrance compounds found in human fat tissue and breast milk is a major concern, as well as contamination of our aquatic life and waterways.

Any politician, junk science reporter, or doctor who tries to defend the fragrance industry, may have ties with the industry or the Chemical Manufacturing Association (CMA). The fragrance industry is a multi-billion dollar industry, and money speaks volumes.

What may seem pleasing to your senses may not be pleasing to others. More importantly, consider our children, as their brains are still developing. Think about our unborn children, as they are at risk for fetal abnormalities. Consider the alarming increase of asthma, MCS, breast cancers, other cancers, and neurological diseases. They are *all* on the rise.

Man has created a toxic mess that I do not believe will be cleaned up in our lifetime, nor in our children's lifetime, nor in our grandchildren's lifetime—possibly, it will never be cleaned up. Millions of people's lives have been ruined by ubiquitous toxic chemicals.

It seems apparent that the toxicity of perfumes is quickly taking a toll on people's health. Material Safety Data Sheets do not lie.

Note that our government claims to be anti-drug/anti-narcotic.

I feel it is unconscionable for our government to keep secrets from the people whom they are elected by, in order to serve and protect.

The Fragrance Foundation, created in 1949, is the arm of the fragrance industry. The industry's biggest *new* thing is retooling classics. The American public makes up the largest fragrance market in the world. [30]

To learn more about the dangers of synthetic fragrances, please read the websites I've provided and help spread the word. The websites contain in-depth information—an abundance of information I couldn't possibly begin to cover in one simple book. Get involved! Your life or that of your loved ones may depend on it.

I hope to have shed "the light of awareness" on the dark side of perfumes.

ADDITIONAL BOOKS OF INTEREST

Chemical Injury and the Court:
A Litigation Guide for Clients and Their Attorneys
Author: Linda Price King
Forward by Will Collette

Multiple Chemical Sensitivity
A Survival Guide
Pamela Reed Gibson, Ph.D.

Casualties of Progress
Personal Histories from the Chemically Sensitive
By Alison Johnson

Fragrance and Health
By Louise Kosta

Chemical Exposures:
Low Levels and High Stakes
By Nicholas A. Ashford, Ph.D. and Claudia S. Miller, M.D.

Is This Your Child?
By Doris Rapp, M.D.
A review of the multitude of environmental influences of your child's behavior and ability to learn.

Chemical Sensitivity, Vols. 1, 2, and 3
By Will J. Rea, M.D.
Documentation of Dr. Rea's findings regarding chemical sensitivity, based on his experience with 20,000 patients. Aimed at the medical field.

Staying Well in a Toxic World
By Lynn Lawson
Understanding Environmental Illness
Multiple Chemical Sensitivities
Chemical Injuries
Sick Building Syndrome

Drop-Dead Gorgeous
Protecting Yourself from the Hidden Dangers of Cosmetics
By Kim Erickson
Forward by Samuel S. Epstein, M.D., author of *The Safe Shopper's Bible*

APPENDIX

Resource List for Organizations and Institutions

CANCER RESEARCH CENTER OF AMERICA, INC.
James W. Coleman, Ph.D., President/CEO
8622 Blackpool Drive
Louisville, KY USA 40222-5667
Phone: (502) 339-1282
Fax: (502) 339-1134
E-mail: mailto:info@CancerResearchAmerica.org

CANCER PREVENTION COALITION, INC.
Samuel S. Epstein, M.D.
University of Illinois School of Public Health
2121 West Taylor Street
Chicago, IL 60612
Phone: (312) 996-2297
Fax: (312) 413-9898
E-mail: mailto:epstein@uic.edu

ANDERSON LABORATORIES, INC.
Julius H. Anderson, M.D., Ph.D., Vice President
Rosalind C. Anderson, Ph.D.
P.O. Box 323
773 Main Street
West Hartford, VT 05084
Phone: (802) 295-7344
Website: http://www.andersonlaboratories.com/

ENVIRONMENTAL HEALTH NETWORK
P.O. Box 1155
Larkspur, CA 94977-1155
Phone: (415) 541-5075
Website: http://users.lmi.net/~wilworks/ehnindex.htm

CHEMICAL INJURY INFORMATION NETWORK (CIIN)
P.O. Box 301
White Sulphur Springs, MT 59645
Phone: (406) 547-2455
Fax: (406) 547-2455
E-mail: mailto:chemicalinjury@ciin.org
Website: http://www.ciin.org/

HUMAN ECOLOGY ACTION LEAGUE, INC.
P.O. Box 29629
Atlanta, GA 30359-0629
Phone: (404) 248-1898
Fax: (404) 248-0162
E-mail: mailto:HEALNatnl@aol.com
Website: http://www.members.aol.com/HEALNatnl/index.html

MASSACHUSETTS ASSOCIATION FOR THE CHEMICALLY INJURED, INC.
P.O. Box 754
Andover, MA 01810
Phone: (978) 681-5117
Fax: (978) 686-0745
E-mail: mailto:MACIMCS@aol.com

MCS: HEALTH AND ENVIRONMENT
2549 Waukegan Road, PMB 162
Bannockburn, IL 60015
Phone: (847) 604-2690
E-mail: mailto:CanaryNews@mcsHealth.Environ.org
Website: http://www.mcshealthenviron.org/

OHIO NETWORK FOR THE CHEMICALLY INJURED
P.O. Box 44129
Phone: (440) 845-1888
Website: http://www.ncchem.com/ONFCI/

ENVIRONMENTAL RESEARCH FOUNDATION
P.O. Box 5036
Annapolis, MD 21403
Fax: (410) 263-8944
E-mail: mailto:erf@rachel.org

NATIONAL CENTER FOR ENVIRONMENTAL HEALTH STRATEGIES
1100 Rural Avenue
Voorhees, NJ 08043
Phone: (856) 429-5358
E-mail: mailto:info@ncehs.org
Website: http://www.ncehs.org/

ENVIRONMENTAL ILLNESS SOCIETY OF CANADA
536 Dovercourt Avenue
Ottawa, Ontario K2A OT9
Phone: (613) 728-9493
Fax: (613) 728-1757
E-mail: mailto:eisc@eisc.ca
Website: http://www.eisc.ca/index1.html

CITIZENS FOR A SAFE LEARNING ENVIRONMENT
287 Lacewood Drive, Unit 103, Suite 178
Halifax, Nova Scotia, B3M 3Y7
902/ 457-3002, 861-1851, 443-6237, 885-2395
E-mail: mailto:am077@chebucto.ns.ca

RESOURCES

1. U.S. Environmental Protection Agency (EPA). *Common Contaminants and Their Health Effects.*
   <http://epa.gov/superfund/programs/er/hazsubs/sources.htm>
   (Referenced: 2002, May.)

   EPA Chemical References Index. *Envirofacts Master Chemical Integrator (EMCI).*
   <http://www.epa.gov/superfund/sites/> (Referenced: 2002, May.)

2. Kendall, Julia. *Making Sense of Scents.*
   <http://www.ourlittleplace.com/scents.html> (Referenced: 2002, July.)

3. Environmental Protection Agency. *Identification of Polar Volatile Organic Compounds in Consumer Products and Common Microenvironments.* Report No. EPA/600/D-91/074, Paper #A312, March 1, 1991.

4. National Headache Foundation. *NHF Headache Facts.*
   <http://www.headaches.org/> (Referenced: 2003, May.)

5. American P.I.E. (American Public Information on the Internet). *Eco Alert: Nonsense Scents,* Jan. 23, 2002.
   <http://www.americanpie.org/> (Referenced: 2002, July.)

6. U.S. National Library of Medicine. *Five Prevalence Surveys on MCS.* (Four of the five citations: <http://www.nlm.nih.gov/> medical journal search).

   One unpublished survey from New Mexico Dept. of Health. (Referenced 2002, Feb.)

7. Nowakowski, Beata, Senior Editor. "Examples of Accommodation: When Fragrances Are Toxic." *EMonthly,* CCH Canadian Limited, Sept. 2001.
<http://www.ca.cch.com/emonthly/sept/hr/index1.asp>
(Referenced: 2002, July.)

8. Greenberg, Larry M. "One City Turns Up Its Nose Against the Use of Perfumes." *The Wall Street Journal,* July 28, 1999. Copyright 1999.

9. Bridges, Betty, RN. *Safe Notification Information for Fragrances – Bill Status & Summary.*
<http://www.fpinva.org.activism__advocacy.HR1947.status.htm>
(Referenced: 2002, March.)

10. "Perfume Triggers Reaction Via The Eyes." *Allergy,* 1999; 54:495–499. New York, Jun. 18, 1999. Copyright 1999, Reuters Ltd.

11. "Everyday Chemicals—Are They Making You Sick?" *Awake Magazine,* Aug. 8, 2000, 3–10.

12. Coleman, James W., Ph.D. *Cosmetics Linked to the Causes of Breast Cancer and Fatal Breast Cancer.*
<http://www.CancerResearchAmerica.org/edu.html> (Referenced: 2002, August.)

13. Excerpts from Moser, Sandra L., Citizens for a Safe Learning Environment. *Fragrance Chemicals As Toxic Substances.*
<http://www.chebucto.ns.ca/Education/CASLE/fragrance.html>
(Referenced: 2002, May.)

14. Woods, Michael. "Synthetic Musk Linked to Environmental Risk." *The Toledo Blade News,* March 24, 1999. Copyright 1999–2003.
<http://www.toledoblade.com/> (Referenced: 2003, July.)

15. Excerpts from Anderson, Julius H., M.D., Ph.D. and Anderson, Rosalind C., Ph.D. *Acute Toxic Effects of Fragranced Products.* Submitted for publication Nov. 14, 1996; revised; accepted for publication May 25, 1997. Archives of Environmental Health, 1998 Mar–Apr; Vol. 53, pages 138–46.
<http://www.andersonlaboratories.com/> (Referenced: 1999, July.)

16. Excerpts from Anderson, Julius H., M.D., Ph.D. and Anderson, Rosalind C., Ph.D. *Toxic Effects of Air Freshener Emissions.* Submitted for publication July 23, 1996; revised; accepted for publication Jan. 16, 1997. Archives of Environmental Health, 1997 Nov–Dec; Vol. 52, pages 433–441.
<http://www.andersonlaboratories.com/> (Referenced: 1999, July.)

17. Department of Health, Education, and Welfare, National Technical Information Services (NTIS). *Health Hazard Evaluation Report HETA 91-026-2257.* Sept. 92, 22p., Order #PB94165123. Phone: 1-800-553-NTIS (U.S. customers); (703) 605-6000 (other countries).

18. Jordan, Sandra. "Note from Nova Scotia: Perfume stinks." *The Detroit News,* London Observer Service, 6/7/00. Copyright 2000. <http://detnews.com/2000/religion/0006/13/06070003.htm> (Referenced: 2002, July.)

19. Bridges, Betty, RN. *The "REAL" facts the industry does not want you to know.* (A rebuttal to the fragrance industry's publicity campaign.)
<http://www.fpinva.org/activist_advocacy.halifax.rebuttal_press_release.htm> (Referenced: 2002, Aug.)

20. Environmental Illness Society of Canada (EISC). *Dangers of Fragranced Candles.*
<http://www.eisc.ca/candles.htm> (Referenced: 2002, July.)

21. Flanders, Cathy. *Candles, Toxic Emissions & Property Damage.* <http://www.fpinva.org/array_of_products.candles.flanders.htm> (Referenced: 2002, July.)

22. Smarr, Pamela. "Healing Our Bodies, Healing the Earth." *Response Magazine.*
<http://gbgm-umc.org/Response/articles/health.html> (Referenced: 2002, July.)

23. Montague, Peter. "Making the Movement Visible (Money Rules)." *Rachel's Environment & Health News,* article #680, New Brunswick, N.J.: Environmental Research Foundation, Dec. 16, 1999.
<http://www.rachel.org/> (Referenced: 2000, Feb.)

24. Bridges, Betty, RN. *Fragrance Chemicals in Tobacco Products.*
    <http://www.fpinva.org/Array/array_of_products.tobacco.htm>
    (Referenced: 2002, May.)

    Indiana Prevention Resource Center. *Additives found in American Cigarettes.*
    <http://www.drugs.indiana.edu/druginfo/additives.html>
    (Referenced: 2002, May.)

25. Foster, Dick. "Illnesses at Army building caused by air freshener." *Rocky Mountain News,* Colorado Springs, 11 February 2000, pg. A5.

26. Powell, Steve. "Students get suspension for cologne in classroom." *Everett Heraldnet,* Marysville, March 21, 2000.
    <http://www.heraldnet.com/Stories/00/3/21/12389861.htm> (Referenced: 2002, June.)

27. The *Los Angeles Times.* "Fragrant freeway stunk 'reeks' havoc on traffic." *Rocky Mountain News,* Leon, Mexico, 29 June 2000, pg. A26.

28. World Briefing. "19 dead from drinking cologne." *Rocky Mountain News,* Riyadh, Saudi Arabia, 10 June 2002, pg. A29.

29. Associated Press. "Florida woman charged with using perfume to hurt husband." *San Francisco Chronicle,* May 10, 2003.
    <http://www.sfgate.com/cgibin/article.cgi?file=/news/archive/2003/05/10/national2311EDT0662.DTL> (Referenced: 2003, May.)

30. Critchell, Samantha. "Classics lite: The scents of summer waft this way." *Rocky Mountain News,* 1 May 2003, Spotlight, pg. 5.

About the Author

Connie Pitts is a wife, mother of two grown daughters, and adores her two young granddaughters. She resides in Colorado, enjoying the majestic beauty of the mountains. As a young adult, she was diagnosed with Fibromyalgia, which eventually led to disability. Being a former perfume user, she is also plagued with a secondary disabling condition, Multiple Chemical Sensitivities (MCS). Searching for answers to her perfume sensitivities, she learned shocking information. Connie is a first time author, compelled by a strong sense of commitment to share her newfound knowledge with other people, as she believes everyone has a right and a need to know the truth.

Printed in Great Britain
by Amazon.co.uk, Ltd.,
Marston Gate.